# Nonsurgical Biliary Drainage

Edited by
M. Classen, J. Geenen and K. Kawai

With 49 Figures

Springer-Verlag
Berlin Heidelberg New York Tokyo 1984

Prof. Dr. med. M. Classen
Abteilung für Gastroenterologie
Zentrum der Inneren Medizin
Universitätsklinikum
Theodor-Stern-Kai 7
D-6000 Frankfurt/M 70, FRG

Dr. J. E. Geenen, M. D.
Clinical Professor of Medicine,
Medical College of Wisconsin,
Director Digestive Disease Center,
St. Luke's Hospital,
Racine, Wisconsin, USA

Prof. K. Kawai, M. D.
Dept. of Preventive Medicine,
Kyoto Prefectural University of Medicine,
Kawaramachi-Hiroloji,
Kyoto, Japan

ISBN-13: 978-3-642-68727-3 e-ISBN-13: 978-3-642-68725-9
DOI: 10.1007/978-3-642-68725-9

Library of Congress Cataloging in Publication Data. Nonsurgical biliary drainage. 1. Bile-ducts-Obstructions-Treatment. 2. Bile-ducts-Catheterization. I. Classen, M. II. Geenen, J. E. III. Kawai, K. [DNLM: 1. Cholestasis-Diagnosis. 2. Cholestasis-Therapy. 3. Drainage-Methods. WI 703 N814] RC851.N58 1984 616.3'65'06 84-5536



Printing and Bookbinding: Brühlsche Universitätsdruckerei, Giessen
2121/3020-543210

# Preface

Mechanical blockage of the common bile duct is a condition that has to be treated by surgery. While this statement is still valid today, it is incomplete.

The immense progress in endoscopy and in X-ray techniques has greatly improved diagnosis and the possibilities of differentiating biliary malignancies. This has been possible due to the development of direct cholangiography with the instillation of contrast medium by the percutaneous transhepatic approach, and of endoscopy via the papilla of Vater (papilla duodeni major).

Applying both methods leads to the identification of blockages in 98 of 100 cases. Lately, by using this combined method, it has become possible to introduce flexible catheters into the common bile duct to drain off bile. This method makes it possible to treat the already existing blockage and to obtain pure bile for bacteriological and antibiotic study. Moreover, prostheses can be implanted into the bile duct by the endoscopic or the percutaneous transhepatic approach to guide the interrupted bile flow into the intestine. This extends the lifespan of some inoperable patients and improves the quality of their lives.

Experts from various medical disciplines have contributed to this book on nonsurgical biliary drainage, published 100 years after C. Langenbeck performed the first cholecystectomy.

Meinhard Classen
Joe Geenen
Keiichi Kawai

# Contents

# List of Contributors

*B. Arnesjö*
Department of Surgery, Haukeland Hospital, University of Bergen, Bergen, Norway

*K. Bakkevold*
Department of Surgery, Haukeland Hospital, University of Bergen, Bergen, Norway

*H. Baumgärtel*
Zentrum der Inneren Medizin, Universitätsklinikum, Theodor-Stern-Kai 7, D-6000 Frankfurt/M, FRG

*D. Brinkley*
Department of Diagnostic Radiology, Radiotherapy, and Oncology, King's College Hospital and Medical School, Denmark Hill, London SE 5, UK

*F. Burcharth*
Department of Surgical Gastroenterology, D 106 Herlev University Hospital, 2730 Herlev, Copenhagen, Denmark

*P. B. Cotton*
Consultant Physician, The Middlesex Hospital, Mortimer Street, London W1 N8AA, UK

*J. L. Dawson*
The Liver Unit, King's College Hospital and Medical School, Denmark Hill, London SE 5, UK

*J. S. Dooley*
Department of Health & Human Services, National Institutes of Health, Bethesda, Maryland 20205, USA

*M. S. Fletcher*
Department of Surgery, King's College Hospital and Medical School, Denmark Hill, London SE 5, UK

*J. E. Geenen*
Medical College of Wisconsin, Director Digestive Disease Center, St. Luke's Hospital, Racine, Wisconsin, USA

*F. Hagenmüller*
Abt. für Gastroenterologie, Zentrum der Inneren Medizin, Universitätsklinikum, Theodor-Stern-Kai 7, D-6000 Frankfurt/M, FRG

*A. R. W. Hatfield*
Academic Unit of Gastroenterology, The London Hospital Whitechapel, London E1, UK

*E. B. Helm*
Zentrum der Inneren Medizin, Universitätsklinikum, Theodor-Stern-Kai 7, D-6000 Frankfurt/M, FRG

*A. F. Hofmann*
Division of Gastroenterology, Department of Medicine, UCSD Medical Center, 225 Dickinson Street, San Diego, CA 92103, USA

*J. Hoevels*
Institut für Klinische Radiologie, Klinikum der Stadt Mannheim, D-6800 Mannheim, FRG

*M. Hölscher*
Chirurgische Klinik und Poliklinik rechts der Isar der Technischen Universität München, Ismaninger Straße 22, D-8000 München, FRG

*K. Huibregtse*
University of Amsterdam, Department of Internal Medicine, Division of Gastroenterology, Wilhelmina Gasthuis, Amsterdam, The Netherlands

*T. Imamura*
Second Department of Surgery, Kurume University School of Medicine, Kurume 830, Japan

*T. Isomura*
Second Department of Surgery, Kurume University School of Medicine, Kurume 830, Japan

*I. Klempa*
Allgemein-Chirurgische Klinik, Zentralkrankenhaus, St.-Jürgen-Straße, D-2800 Bremen, FRG

*M. Koga*
Second Department of Surgery, Kurume University School of Medicine, Kurume 830, Japan

*U. Leuschner*
Zentrum der Inneren Medizin, Universitätsklinikum, Theodor-Stern-Kai 7, D-6000 Frankfurt/M, FRG

*A. Lunderquist*
Department of Diagnostic Radiology, University Hospital, Lund, Sweden

*T. Nakayama*
Second Department of Surgery, Kurume University School of Medicine, Kurume 830, Japan

H. Nunnerley
Department of Diagnostic Radiology, King's College Hospital and Medical School, Denmark Hill, London SE 5, UK

*J. F. Riemann*
Medizinische Klinik mit Poliklinik der Universität Erlangen, Krankenhausstr. 12, D-8520 Erlangen, FRG

*H. Saitsu*
Second Department of Surgery, Kurume University School of Medicine, Kurume 830, Japan

*M. Sata*
Second Department of Surgery, Kurume University School of Medicine, Kurume 830, Japan

*J. R. Siewert*
Chirurgische Klinik und Poliklinik rechts der Isar der Technischen Universität München, Ismaninger Straße 22, D-8000 München, FRG

*N. Soehendra*

Abteilung für Abdominalchirurgie, Universitätskrankenhaus Eppendorf, Martinistr. 52, D-2000 Hamburg 20, FRG

*W. Stille*

Zentrum der Inneren Medizin, Universitätsklinikum, Theodor-Stern-Kai 7, D-6000 Frankfurt/M, FRG

*T. Tanaka*

Second Department of Surgery, Kurume University School of Medicine, Kurume 830, Japan

*J. Terblanche*

Department of Surgery, University of Cape Town Medical School, Observatory 7925, Cape Town, South Africa

*K. Weinbren*

Royal Postgraduate Medical School, London

*R. Williams*

Department of Radiotherapy and Oncology, King's College Hospital and Medical School, Denmark Hill, London SE 5, UK

*D. Wurbs*

I. Medizinische Abteilung für Gastroenterologie, Allgemeines Krankenhaus Barmbek, Rübenkamp 148, D-2000 Hamburg 60, FRG

*M. Yano*

Second Department of Surgery, Kurume University School of Medicine, Kurume 830, Japan

*S. Yokomizo*

Second Department of Surgery, Kurume University School of Medicine, Kurume 830, Japan

# I. Obstruction of the Bile Ducts: Pathology and Surgery

# 1 Pathology

*K. Weinbren*

Changes in the human liver in obstructive jaundice involve the whole biliary tree and in addition hepatocytes and macrophages.

The changes include several that in combination are good indicators of the major underlying structural abnormalities, and occasional changes that are pathognomonic. The possible reactions of cells making up the liver are limited and therefore there is considerable overlap between different conditions. For example, canalicular stasis is reported in over 80% of biopsy specimens taken from patients suffering from viral hepatitis, ductal proliferation occurs in several conditions other than large-duct obstruction, e.g., α-anti-trypsin deficiency, small biliary necroses are present in drug toxicity, and portal neutrophil accumulations are regularly present in alcoholic hepatitis and sometimes in patients suffering from ulcerative colitis.

The changes associated with large-duct obstruction are familiar, but the mechanisms are not fully understood. Even that of canalicular stasis, without which a diagnosis of structural obstructive jaundice is difficult to sustain, has not yet been worked out. It is still not known, why the pigment precipitates are found predominantly perivenously and whether there is always canaliculolymphatic leakage.

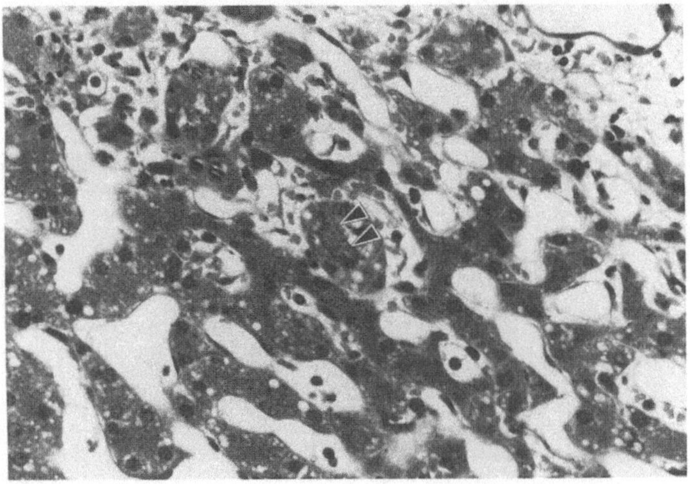

**Fig. 1.** Intracanalicular inspissate in duct obstruction *(arrow)*. H & E, ×400

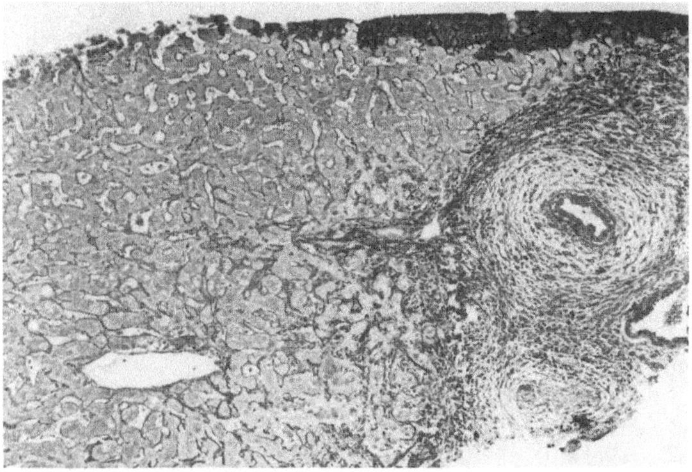

**Fig. 2.** Periductal fibrosis in liver with long-standing duct obstruction. Gordon and Sweet reticulin impregnation, ×60

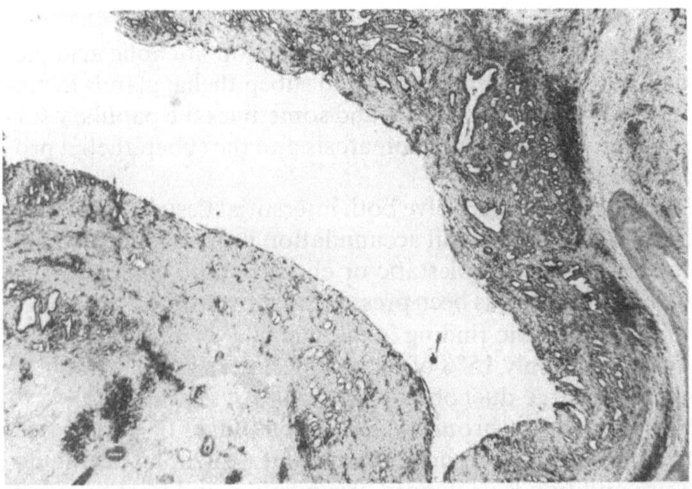

**Fig. 3.** Section of duct with chronic pyogenic cholangitis, showing severe proliferation of subepithelial mucous glands. H & E, ×60

The second major change in duct obstruction involves proliferation of components of the biliary tree. Canaliculi do not proliferate, though they dilate, but marginal ducts with recognizable lumina are found to be increased in number on section. This probably reflects tortuosity, but also an increased number of cells. Again, this is not unique of duct obstruction, occurring very frequently in conditions in which hepatocytes are damaged, and there seems to be an inverse relationship between hepatocyte proliferation and ductal proliferation. Sometimes ductal proliferation is so exuberant after hepatocyte destruction that cholangiocarcinoma is simulated. The mechanism of marginal duct proliferation is not

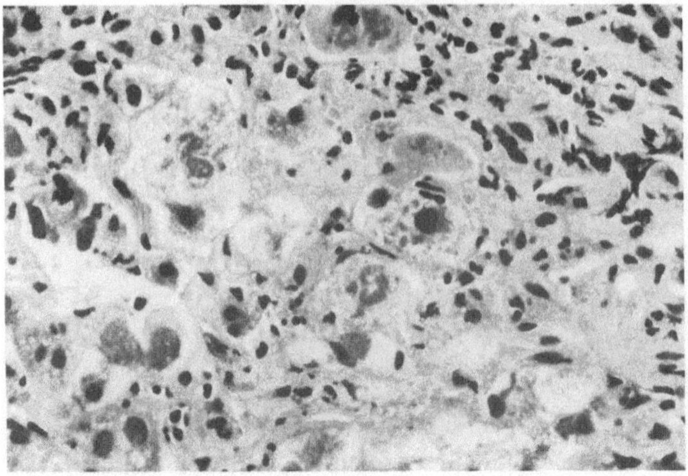

**Fig. 4.** Periportal liver cells containing hyalin (copper-binding protein) in severe long-standing obstructive jaundice. H & E, ×600

known, and speculation has included the proliferogenic action of cholic acid metabolites. Proliferation of both surface epithelium and subepithelial glands in major ducts is a regular finding in duct obstruction, and sometimes the papillary surface change has excited the suspicion of papillomatosis and the subepithelial proliferations of invasive neoplasm.

Major accompanying abnormalities involve both interstitial tissue and hepatocytes, the portal tract edema and neutrophil accumulation probably occurring in most cases and hepatocyte so-called cholestatic or cholate-static changes being present in patients in whom jaundice has been present for some weeks.

The one genuinely pathognomonic finding is the bile lake or Charcot–Gombault necrosis, which is found in only 15% of biopsy specimens but has not been found in conditions other than large-duct obstruction.

The evolution of the changes with chronicity is largely as might be anticipated. Although the ultimate stimulus for the portal edema and neutrophil accumulation is not defined, if this condition is prolonged organization and fibrosis ensue, so that portal fibrosis is a regular accompaniment of long-standing obstruction. True cirrhosis, with hyperplastic nodules in which vascular relations are not maintained, was recognized by Gibson and Robertson in 1939 to be extremely rare (occurring in fewer than 10% of cases) and to require an inordinately prolonged period of obstruction.

Many of the changes, however, vary with the cause of the obstruction. In those associated with extensive cholangitis, such as pyogenic cholangitis, intermittent lesions, and postoperative complications, the acute exudate is often associated with an accumulation of lymphocytes and these may form focal collections. This can sometimes simulate the inflammatory component of primary biliary cirrhosis, but the ductal changes serve to distinguish these two in most instances. However, the fibrosis which is often present may compromise bile ducts, which on clinical

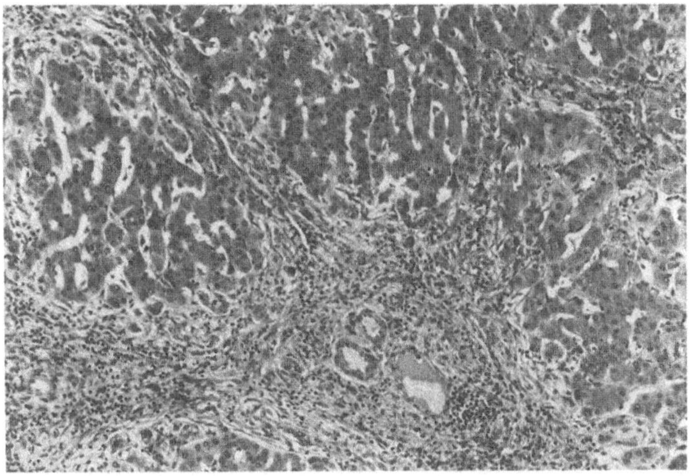

**Fig. 5.** Hepatocyte hyperplasia with formation of 2-cell-thick plates and accumulation of lymphocytes with marginal duct proliferation. H & E, × 150

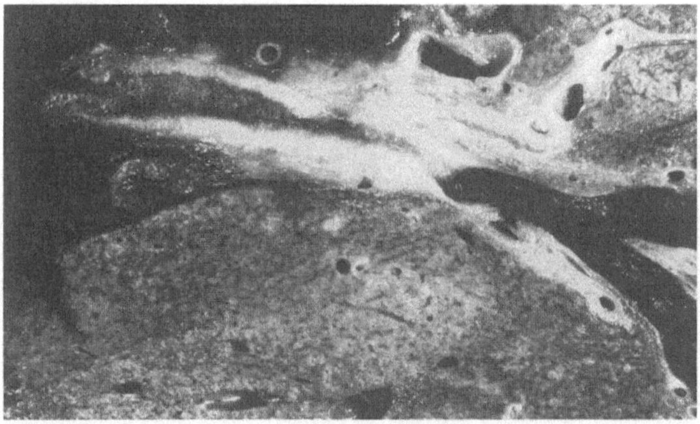

**Fig. 6.** Sclerosing carcinoma of bile duct causing obstructive jaundice

examination or imaging may lead to the diagnosis of primary sclerosing cholangitis.

True sclerosing cholangitis, in our experience, involves the replacement of ducts by whorls of fibrous tissue, and lumina are invariably compromised with evidence of epithelial destruction. This lesion is distinct from pericholangitis and is sometimes complicated by the development of cholangiocarcinoma.

The question of cholangiocarcinoma is one that is attracting increasing interest, although it accounts for fewer than 10% of all cases of hepatocellular carcinoma in the West, because of major advances in and options for surgery.

At The Royal Postgraduate Medical School at Hammersmith in London, a large number of patients suffering from cholangiocarcinoma have been referred

**Table 1.** Numbers of patients compared in attempt to define diagnostic criteria

| Condition | Biliary tumors | Obstructive jaundice | Other intrahepatic tumors |
|---|---|---|---|
| Number of patients | 33 | 12 | 13 |

**Table 2.** Areas of liver from which material was derived

| Area | No. of specimens |
|---|---|
| Diffuse hepatic | 4 |
| Confluence | 10 |
| R. hepatic | 4 |
| L. hepatic | 2 |
| CHD | 3 |
| CBD | 3 |
| Ampullary and peripapillary | 7 |

**Table 3.** Gross appearance of tumors at different sites within the liver

| Site (no.) | Annular sclerosing | Nodular | Papillary |
|---|---|---|---|
| Upper (23) | 21 | 0 | 2 |
| Mid (3) | 0 | 3 | 0 |
| Lower (7) | 0 | 0 | 7 |

over the past 3 years. In view of the importance of avoiding more than one procedure we have tried to define diagnostic criteria by examining all resected specimens and comparing the findings with groups of controls. In this way, tissue samples from some 33 patients with cholangiocarcinoma have been compared with 12 with duct obstruction not due to cholangiocarcinoma and 13 with other tumors in the liver (Table 1). The tissue samples were all prepared in a standard way and assessed by one of two appropriate procedures. The material was derived from all areas of the liver up to the ampulla (Table 2). The findings were of interest in that for the most part, characteristic tumors occupied characteristic sites, the exceptions being special cases, such as papillomatosis or cystic disease (Table 3); and the relevant microscopical characteristics of tumors included mucin production as the main one in all cases (Table 4). Certain changes were common to

**Table 4.** Microscopical features of the different conditions considered

| Condition (No. of cases) Characteristic | Biliary tumors (33) | Obstructive jaundice (12) | Other tumors (13) |
|---|---|---|---|
| Mucin production | 33 | – | 8 |
| Presence of free mucin | 16 | 0 | 0 |
| Cellular variability | 10 | 0 | 0 |
| Neural involvement | 19 | 0 | 0 |
| Fibrosis of intra-vascular tumor | 1 | 0 | 0 |

neoplastic and nonneoplastic duct obstruction, such as subepithelial glandular proliferation; certain changes were highly suggestive of neoplasm, such as variable cytology within the same lining epithelium and subepithelial tumor growth; and some conditions indicated such chronicity that they were unlikely to be associated with neoplasia, such as copper-protein complex accumulation and the development of true cirrhosis.

Among the many other points which emerged from the study, one striking feature was the severe fibrosis, which rendered the limits of the tumor difficult to define and which occurred even during venous invasion, which may be why this tumor metastasizes so infrequently; and although cholangitis and abscess formation are not thought to be common in cholangiocarcinoma, they were in fact noted in most instances when patients had had previous operations. This means, of course, that they are frequently present by the time patients with cholangiocarcinoma are referred to centers with a special interest in this clinical problem.

# 2 Indications for Surgery in Benign and Malignant Bile Duct Obstruction

*J. R. Siewert and M. Hölscher*

Cancer statistics suggest that there will be 13,000 new cases of cancer involving the liver and biliary passages in any one year in the United States of America (Tompkins et al. 1981). This amounts to about 7% of all new cancers of the digestive tract per year. On the other hand, a high incidence of gallstone disease is responsible for about 300,000 operations on the biliary tract each year. The coincidence of common bile duct stones and earlier cholecystectomy varies between 5% and 25%. In view of these figures, physicians and surgeons anticipate that the problem of obstruction of the common bile duct will arise quite often.

## Definition

By obstruction of the common bile duct we understand all blockages caused by stenoses or strictures, by intraluminal stones, etc., or by a combination of both, regardless of extent and localization.

## Classification

A pathogenetic classification of common bile duct obstruction is of diagnostic as well as of therapeutic importance (Fig. 1).

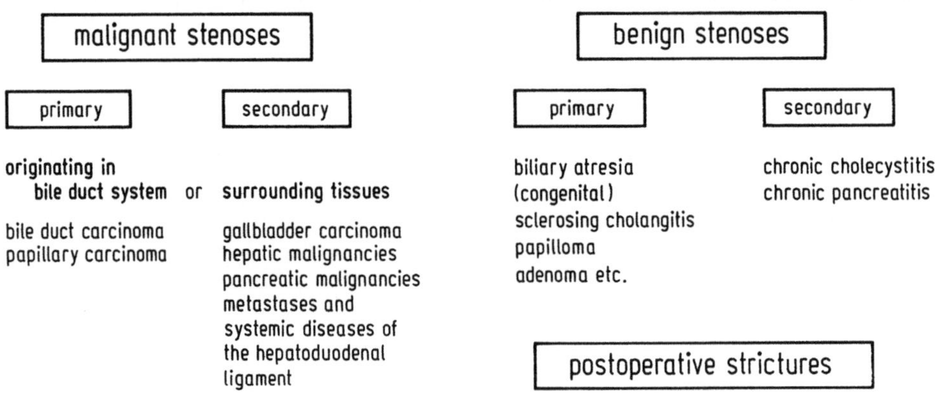


a b

**Fig. 1.** Pathgenetic classification of malignant **a** and benign **b** stenoses or strictures of the common bile duct

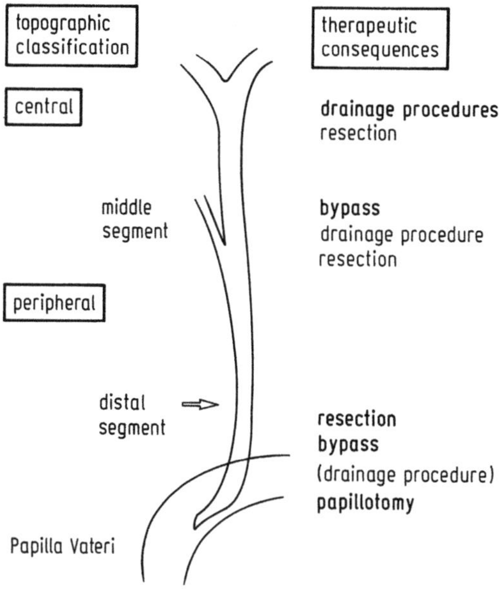


**Fig. 2.** Therapeutic consequences of surgical procedures commonly used in the treatment of common bile duct strictures

Malignant stenoses can be primary, originating in the ductal system, or secondary, deriving from the surrounding tissues such as gallbladder, liver, pancreas, or hepatoduodenal ligament. Usually symptoms of occlusion of the bile duct occur earlier in primary than in secondary malignancies.

Benign stenoses also include primary or secondary pathologic processes, such primary processes as papillomas or adenomas of the ductal system being extremely rare.

These two categories have to be differentiated from postoperative common duct strictures, which are responsible for about 10% of reoperations after biliary surgery but account for up to 96% of benign common bile duct strictures.

In more than 95% of all cases, endoscopic retrograde cholangiography (ERCP) and percutaneous transhepatic cholangiography (PTC) reveal a localization, extent, and kind of obstruction that are pathognomonic. Multiple and solitary lesions can be differentiated. The classification of bile duct obstruction by localization – central, proximal, or distal peripheral occlusion – is nowadays important not only for surgical therapy but also for nonoperative drainage procedures. The "therapeutic consequences" cited in Fig. 2 refer to surgical procedures frequently used in the treatment of common bile duct strictures.

Morphologic, functional, and the most important clinical criteria can be used to differentiate between compensated and decompensated bile duct obstruction (Table 1). Prestenotic dilatation, jaundice, and clinical symptoms such as colic attacks and fever and chills indicate decompensated bile duct obstruction.

Pathogenetic differentiation, localization, differentiation between compensated and decompensated bile duct obstruction, and the availability of a variety of surgical and nonsurgical methods of treatment demand a high degree of discrimination in diagnosis and selection of therapy.

**Table 1.** Differentation between compensated and decompensated bile duct obstruction by application of varios criteria

| Criteria | Compensated | Decompensated |
|---|---|---|
| Morphological | Non-dilated ducts | Prestenotic *dilatation* |
| Functional | Normal liver function and enzymes, or mild elevation of AP; LAP | Subclinical → clinical *Jaundice* |
| Clinical | No complications | *Colic attacks* (stone formation)<br>*Fever* (cholangitis, abscess)<br>*Liver insufficiency* (cirrhosis) |

## Indications

It is rare for emergency operations to have to be performed; indications are intra-abdominal perforation, diffuse peritonitis, intra-abdominal abscess formation, and even ileus coexisting with, or causally connected with, common bile duct obstruction. Generally there is enough time to establish the diagnosis of bile duct obstruction.

Decompensated obstructions are always an indication for therapy, whereas compensated stenoses are an indication only if a malignant lesion cannot be excluded by routine diagnostic procedures. Severe liver cirrhosis can be a contraindication, as can other conditions.

Primary malignant solitary stenoses with a chance of cure by resection are an absolute indication for surgery in theory (Fig. 3). They are located centrally in about 40%–50% of cases, are most often unresectable, and when resected are often incompletely removed. Resection at this level has a higher mortality rate than palliation by an operative drainage procedure using U-T or YT tubes.

Peripheral resection of primary malignant stenoses (Whipple's procedure is considered more often than others) has a higher mortality rate than palliative procedures such as bypass operations. But a 5-year survival rate of 20%–30% can be expected, which justifies major resection for primary distal duct carcinoma, papillary carcinoma, and secondary periampullary carcinoma of the pancreas without any metastases. Other absolute indications for surgery are decompensated benign strictures, whether postoperative, primary or secondary.

The results obtained at the Lahey Clinic from 1940 to 1967 were reported by Warren (1975). This exceptional study of benign strictures indicates a typical location for surgical traumata, and a high rate of clinical decompensation (Table 2). Even though the study presents results collected over a period of nearly 30 years, the frequency of reoperations, success rate, morbidity and mortality illustrate the severe problems encountered in surgical treatment of benign strictures, which are still the same now.

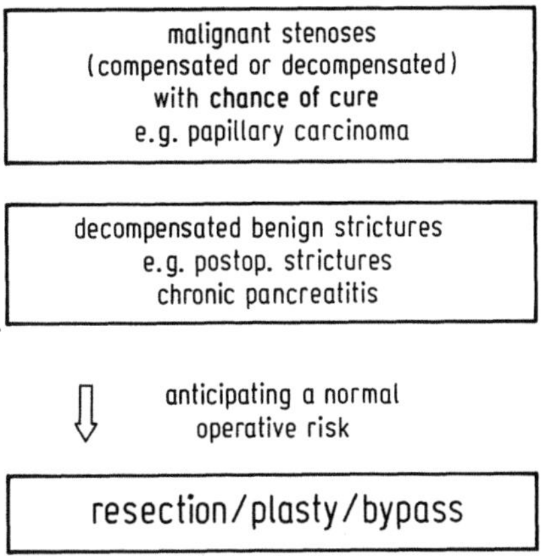


**Fig. 3.** Absolute indications for surgery

**Table 2.** Results of surgery in 987 patients with benign biliary stricture

| | | |
|---|---|---|
| Surgical | Trauma | 97% |
| | Central | 10% |
| Location | Peripheral/ proximal | 89% |
| | Chills and fever | 64% |
| Symptoms | Pain | 49% |
| | Jaundice | 44% |
| Operations | 1.6 patient | |
| Mortality | | 13% |
| Morbidity | | 40% |
| | | Satisfactory |
| End-to-end anastomosis | | 52% |
| Hepaticojejunostomy | | 66% |

Central strictures can often be repaired by Smith's procedure or hepaticojejunostomy. If possible, duct-to-duct anastomosis or plastic repair is preferable to hepaticojejunostomy for repair of peripheral strictures because biliary diversion has some disadvantages (Fig. 4). Cholangitis, stenosis, and the operation's potential ulcerogenicity limit the success of this operation in benign diseases. Absolute indications for major resection or bypass procedures or plastic repair, including anastomoses, are present only if the operative risk is fairly normal.

The indications for surgical therapy are relative in cases of advanced primary malignancy and most cases of secondary malignancy causing bile duct obstruction (Fig. 5). These patients are usually elderly and in poor general health. Drainage procedures and biliary diversions are the procedures of choice.

In primary sclerosing cholangitis with multiple stenoses or in patients with recurrent strictures who have been subjected to frequent surgery, the outcome of surgical treatment is influenced mainly by the quality of the proximal bile duct,

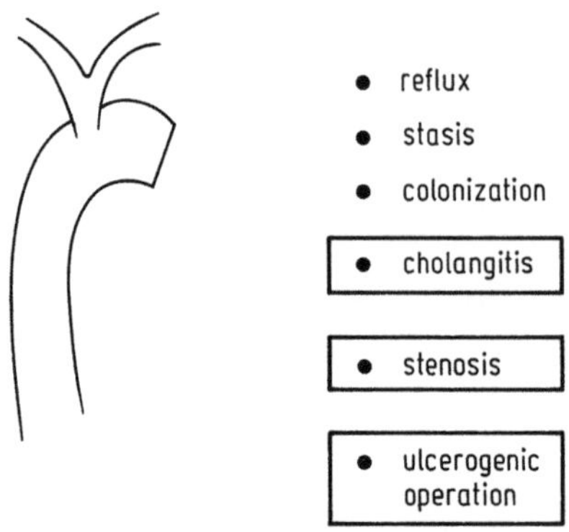


**Fig. 4.** Schematic of hepaticojejunostomy and its disadvantages

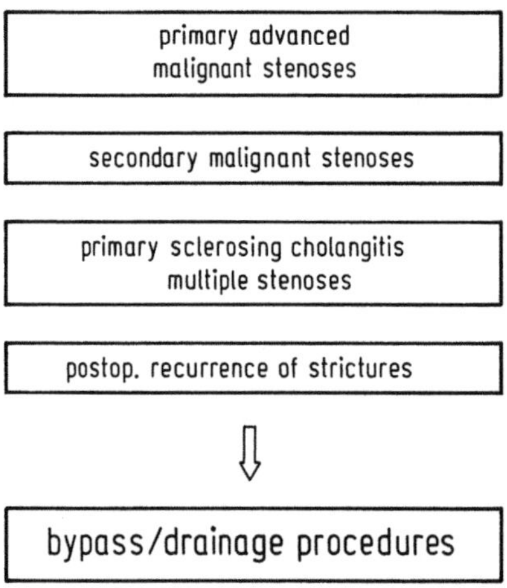


**Fig. 5.** Relative indications for surgical therapy in malignancy causing bile duct obstruction

the presence or absence of inflammation, and the function and pathology of the liver. The prognosis seems to be poor.

In stone disease of common bile ducts, we are anticipating usually gallstones originating in the gallbladder (secondary bile duct stones) whereas primary duct stones develop as a consequence of bile duct strictures or of the presence of foreign bodies such as suture material.

Primary stenosis of the papilla Vateri can be diagnosed only if there is no other pathology of the duodenum, the pancreas or the biliary system. Intraoperative x-ray studies, manometry, and pharmacological tests (cholecystokinin) suggest that the incidence of the combination of bile duct stones with stenosis of the papilla is only about 5%, which is important when the indications for papillotomy are considered.

Surgery for stones in the common bile duct can be vital in the case of perforations of the biliary system, peritonitis, intra-abdominal abscess, ileus, or purulent cholangitis. Biliary pancreatitis does not seem to be an urgent indication for biliary surgery, but if surgery is performed because of pancreatitis, it may be helpful to relieve the bile duct obstruction at the same time.

Decompensated bile duct obstruction by gallstones is always an indication for surgery. For surgical intervention we have to differentiate between patients who have not undergone any biliary surgery and patients who have previously undergone cholecystectomy. The first group, except for older patients in whom surgery involves a high risk, should always be subjected to surgery, especially young patients because, as demonstrated, papillotomy is not necessary in most instances and no good data are available on the outcome of endoscopic papillotomy over a long lifespan. In patients who have undergone cholecystectomy there is a relative indication for surgery, especially in the older age group in whom surgery involves a high risk and in patients who have had multiple operations of the biliary system.

In general, relative indications for surgery in benign and malignant bile duct obstruction are indications for nonoperative treatment.

From the surgical viewpoint, combined procedures such as cholecystectomy and endoscopic papillotomy are indicated because of the risk involved in duodenotomy. Nonoperative drainage is indicated in the presence of decompensated bile duct obstruction by stones or benign or malignant stenoses to achieve preoperative biliary drainage if a major resection is to be performed. We expect lower morbidity and mortality from adequate preoperative drainage procedures.

## References

Tompkins RK, Thomas D, Wile A, Longmire WP (1981) Prognostic factors in bile duct carcinoma. Ann Surg 194:447–455

Warren KW (1975) Diseases of the gallbladder and bile ducts. In: Schiff L (ed) Diseases of the liver, 4th edn. Lippincott, Philadelphia, pp 1278–1335

# 3 Assessment of Resectability

*B. Arnesjö and K. Bakkevold*

Between 70% and 90% of patients with bile duct or pancreatic cancer are incurable, and have tumors that are unresectable by the time they are seen by the surgeon (Cancer Registry of Norway 1980; Cooperman 1981; Ihse 1982). The reason for unresectability or incurability is usually invasion of the main abdominal arteries and veins, or involvement of the tumor at the bifurcation of the hepatic ducts with tumor growth in both lobes of the liver. A significant number of patients also have distant metastases at the time of operation.

Local invasion involving vital blood vessels, tumor manifestations outside the primary site of the lesion, and especially spread to local or distant lymphatic glands and the liver are thus criteria for unresectability – at least if the secondary lesions cannot be removed en bloc with the primary lesion.

The curative procedures to be considered are right or left hepatic lobectomy in patients with hepatic duct cancer occurring proximally in the right or left hepatic ducts. Tumors at the junction of the hepatic ducts and the proximal part of the extrahepatic bile ducts may be removed by local excision, often combined with partial or complete central liver resection and an end-to-end anastomosis of the bile duct or hepaticojejunostomy (Evander et al. 1980; Kune and Sali 1980; Launois et al. 1979; Todoroki et al. 1980; Takasan et al. 1980; Thorbjarnarson 1982). In cases with tumors distal to the cystic duct most surgeons prefer to perform extended pancreaticoduodenal resection or pancreaticoduodenectomy (Howat and Sarles 1979; Moossa et al. 1979; Moossa and Levin 1981; Cooperman 1981; Longmire and Traverso 1981; Hester et al. 1982).

Most of the recorded long-time survivors belong to this latter group. All these advanced surgical procedures can now be performed with reasonable postoperative complication and mortality rates ($< 12\%$ mortality) by experienced surgical teams.

Unfortunately, successful radical excision of the primary lesion is not equivalent to cure in most cases. Less than 30%–35% of patients with bile duct cancer (Thorbjarnarson 1982) and far fewer with pancreatic cancer are alive 5 years after curative resection (Ihse 1982). Palliative excision of such tumors is associated with too high a risk and almost no benefit.

As in many other countries, the extremely poor prognosis in these forms of cancer is well illustrated by the recent survival data published by the Norwegian Cancer Registry in 1980. These data, however, demonstrate a slight increase in the survival rates, especially among women. Although the improvement is slight and its statistical significance is questionable, these better overall results may raise expectations for the future and provide the rationale for a more enthusiastic and aggressive diagnostic and surgical approach to these tumor forms. The factors responsible for this possible improvement are not known, however, and demand detailed prospective studies.

The papers presented during this symposium illustrate the features and manifestations in patients with these serious diseases. In cases with obstruction of the bile duct and cholestasis percutaneous transhepatic or endoscopic internal or external biliary drainage procedures are suggested as preoperative or permanent measures aiming at diagnosis and preoperative preparation in all cases, and perhaps palliation in those with unresectable primary lesions. Cholestasis probably enhances the morbidity and mortality after surgery irrespective of the surgical procedure applied (for references see Nordlander 1982). Thus many investigators have found a higher postoperative complication rate even in unresectable cases subjected to palliative surgical procedures such as bilio-digestive shunts and gastroenterostomy than in connection with nonsurgical drainage procedures. Permanent nonoperative biliary drainage should, however, only be used in patients with conclusive criteria of incurability. In a recent study, Nordlander (1982) has been unable to demonstrate any benefit of preoperative transhepatic biliary drainage in patients with resectable or unresectable obstructive carcinomas of the bile duct and pancreas. Although the results of that study speak in favor of exclusion of biliary drainage as a preparative procedure, results are contradictory. This controversy can only be solved by prospective controlled trials. Until it is proven otherwise we shall continue to believe that preoperative drainage, preferably combined with bile refeeding, is of benefit in resectable cases and a constant method of choice in unresectable cases, in which surgical exploration thus can be avoided.

Recent discussions regarding the field of bile duct and pancreatic carcinomas have mainly focused upon how to diagnose these forms of cancers, preferably at an early stage (Howat and Sarles 1979; Moossa and Levin 1981; Wood 1981; Go et al. 1981). Most clinical investigations have now been replaced by computerized tomography, ultrasonography, ERCP, and/or percutaneous transhepatic cholangiography, sometimes combined with guided percutaneous fine-needle biopsies for histological examination (Tylen et al. 1976). Diagnostic accuracy has reached acceptable levels, whereas the appraisal of resectability usually necessitates complementary investigations such as angiography, percutaneous transhepatic portography, and last but not least, exploratory laparotomy (Wood 1981; Ihse 1982).

Due to the extremely poor prognosis, many surgeons have adopted a defeatist attitude towards these cases and believe there is no point in doing anything but establish palliative biliary drainage (Crile 1970). From being surgical problems, many of these patients have become problems for endoscopists and radiologists and are often offered no chance of curative treatment. The recent possible improvement in the long-term results, however, speaks in favor of surgical exploration in all cases where there are grounds for suspicion or histological verification of carcinoma in this area. An exception might be patients with histologically verified metastases of the liver or other structures fairly far from the primary tumor. In addition, many of these patients are old, not seldom with concomitant complicating diseases making them unsuitable for curative surgery but good candidates for palliative nonsurgical biliary drainage. This latter patient group has not yet been clearly defined.

Many carcinomas, and especially those causing ductal obstruction, are often surrounded by an inflammatory zone, which might mimic an advanced malignant lesion both at work up and peroperatively (Arnesjö et al. 1972; Todoroki et al. 1980). At a thorough surgical dissection, however, such tumors might readily be radically removed despite clinical contraindications. Accordingly, encasement or stenosis of the superior mesenteric vein in cases with periampullary or pancreatic cancer is not rare when the lesion is confined to areas relatively distant from this vessel. Seemingly completely inextirpable tumors at the hepatic duct junction may even fairly often be removed with a reasonable margin after careful hilar dissection.

Some studies have been reported in which specific signs precluding resection have been suggested or postulated. In 1968 Sato et al. (1968) compared clinical features and results of clinical investigations with resectability and prognosis. The predictive value for the judgement of incurability was good for most signs, but not complete. These authors concluded among other things that abdominal pains and signs of general debilitation are signs of unresectability.

In 1973 Tylén and Arnesjö (1973) were able to demonstrate a high rate of unresectability and an extremely poor prognosis in patients with tumor vessels outside the pancreatic parenchyma or encasement of the extrapancreatic main blood vessels. Lack of such angiographic findings meant, besides resectability, much better survival and in some cases apparently cure. That study, however, was an open retrospective study and bias thus cannot be completely excluded. These findings, however, have been confirmed in several recent studies using both angiographic and percutaneous transhepatic portographic techniques (Suzuki et al. 1979; Reichardt and Ihse 1980).

In our opinion, as also demonstrated in several recent reports (Moossa and Levin 1981; Go et al. 1981; Wood 1981), computerized tomography and ultrasonography are not completely reliable methods and may even demonstrate signs of advanced disease in cases where no signs of malignant lesion are found on surgical exploration. Many successful percutaneous, endoscopic, or other forms of preoperative biopsies from a suspected primary tumor in these organs may be indicative, but not conclusive, of the presence of a malignant tumor. Positive histologic diagnosis cannot preclude resection unless biopsies have been obtained from the primary lesion as well as a secondary manifestation of the same tumor. Both ERCP and PTC are good diagnostic tools, especially in combination with percutaneous fine-needle biopsy techniques, but usually of little significance for determination of resectability of a specific tumor (Suzuki et al. 1980).

Overall, we have reached the following conclusions:

1. As the long-term survival in patients with carcinoma of the bile ducts and pancreas seems to be improving, and surgical radical resection is the only known chance of cure, an aggressive surgical approach to the primary tumor seems legitimate.
2. There are no procedures available that can definitely exclude resectability preoperatively, except histologic or cytologic proof of distant metastases from a histologically or cytologically verified primary tumor.
3. Nonoperative internal or external biliary drainage procedures should only be used for preparatory purposes, or perhaps permanently in patients with proven

distant metastases or a general condition making them unsuitable for advanced surgery.
4. The high risk of postoperative complications in patients with jaundice due to unresectable bile duct or pancreatic cancer can perhaps be avoided by using preoperative drainage instead of surgical shunting at and after surgical exploration.
5. This problematic field of gastroenterology and oncology must be investigated in prospective randomized trials.

## References

Arnesjö B, Stormby N, Åkerman M (1972) Cytodiagnosis of pancreatic lesions by means of fine needle biopsy during operation. Acta Chir Scand 138:363–369

Cancer Registry of Norway (1980) Survival of cancer patients. Cases diagnosed in Norway 1968–1975. Oslo pp 204

Cooperman AM (1981 a) Cancer of the ampulla of Vateri, bile duct and duodenum. In: Cooperman AM (ed) Symposium on liver, spleen, and pancreas. Surg Clin North 61(1):99–106

Cooperman AM (1981 b) Cancer of the pancreas: A dilemma of treatment. In: Cooperman AM (ed) Symposium on liver, spleen, and pancreas. Surg Clin North Am 61(1):107–115

Crile G Jr (1970) The advantages of bypass operations over radical pancreaticoduodenectomy in the treatment of pancreatic carcinoma. Surg Gynecol Obstet 130:1049–1053

Evander A, Fredlund P, Hoevels J et al. (1980) Evaluation of aggressive surgery for carcinoma of the extrahepatic bile ducts. Ann Surg 191:23–29

Go VLW, Taylor WF, Di Magno EP (1981) Efforts at early diagnosis of pancreatic cancer. Cancer 47:1698–1703

Hester FP, Cooperman AM, Ahlborn TN, Antinori C (1982) Surgical experience with pancreatic and periampullary cancer. Ann Surg 195:274–281

Howat HT, Sarles H (1979) The exocrine pancreas. Saunders, London, pp 551

Ihse I (1982) Treatment of pancreatic cancer: current status. Scand J Gastroenterol 17:449–453

Kune GA, Sali A (1980) The practice of biliary surgery. Blackwell, Oxford, pp 462

Launois B, Campion JP, Brissot P, Gossclin M (1979) Carcinoma of the hepatic hilus: surgical management and the case for resection. Ann Surg 190:151–157

Longmire WP, Traverso W (1981) The Whipple procedure and other standard operative approaches to pancreatic cancer. Cancer 47:1706–1711

Moossa AR, Levin B (1981) The diagnosis of "early" pancreatic cancer. Cancer 47:1688–1697

Moossa AR, Lewis MH, Mackie CR (1979) Surgical treatment of pancreatic cancer. Mayo Clin Proc 54:468–4

Nordlander A (1982) Studies on biliary drainage of extrahepatic cholestasis in man with special reference to bile acid metabolism. Thesis, Stockholm University

Reichard W, Ihse I (1980) Percutaneous transhepatic portography in pancreatic carcinoma. Acta Radiol [Diagn] (Stockh) 21:579–586

Sato T, Saitoh Y, Koyama R, Watanabe K (1968) Preoperative determination of operability in carcinomas of the pancreas and the periampullary region. Ann Surg 168:876–886

Suzuki T, Imamura M, Tamura K, Sumiyoshi A, Sakanashi S, Nichimura Y, Tobe T (1979) Correlative evaluation of angiography and pancreatoductography in relation to surgery for cancer of the pancreas. Surgery 85:644–651

Suzuki T, Manabe T, Tani T, Tobe T (1980) Angiography and pancreatoductography in resectable carcinoma of the pancreas. Acta Radiol [Diagn] (Stockh) 21:587–591

Takasan H, Kim CJ, Arii S, Takahachi S, Uozumi T, Tobe T, Honjo I (1980) Clinicopathologic study of seventy patients with carcinoma of the biliary tract. Surg Gynecol Obstet 150:721–726

Thorbjarnarson B (1982) Surgery of the biliary tract. 2nd edn. Saunders, Philadelphia, pp 265
Tylén U, Arnesjö B (1973) Resectability and prognosis of carcinoma of the pancreas evaluated by angiography. Scand J Gastroenterol 8:691–697
Tylén U, Arnesjö B, Lindberg LG, Lunderquist A, Åkerman M (1976) Percutaneous biopsy of carcinoma of the pancreas guided by angiography. Surg Gynecol Obstet 142:737–739
Todoroki T, Okaraura T, Fukao K, Nishimura A, Otsu H, Sato H, Iwasaki Y (1980) Gross appearance of carcinoma of the main hepatic duct and its prognosis. Surg Gynecol Obstet 150:33–40
Wood RAB (1981) The diagnosis of pancreatic cancer. In: Lumley, Isp, Craven JL (eds) Surgical review 2. Pituran Medical, London, p 107–117

# II. The Percutaneous Transhepatic Approach

# 4 Techniques of Percutaneous Bile Drainage

*J. Hoevels and A. Lunderquist*

Since Leger and Zara et Arway (1952) described a combination of diagnostic percutaneous transhepatic access to the biliary duct system with preoperative external bile drainage in extrahepatic cholestasis, various techniques have been reported for biliary decompression by percutaneous transhepatic intubation of the bile ducts. Initially only external drainage of the obstructed biliary ducts was performed (Ahnlund and Morales 1963; Kaude et al. 1969; Takada et al. 1976; Burcharth and Nielbo 1976; Tylén et al. 1977; Mori et al. 1977). In recent years the therapeutic efficacy of bile drainage via a nonsurgically introduced catheter has been further improved. Manipulation of a guide wire and a drainage catheter through the obstructing lesion allows both internal and external bile flow (Molnar and Stockum 1974; Takada et al. 1977; Nakayama et al. 1978; Hoevels et al. 1978a; Ring et al. 1978; Rupp et al. 1979; Ferrucci et al. 1980; Berquist et al. 1981; McLean et al. 1982; Mueller et al. 1982a).

Percutaneous transhepatic cholangiography (PTC) and percutaneous transhepatic biliary drainage are performed in two stages, necessitating two separate punctures of the intrahepatic biliary tract. Fine-needle PTC as the first step facilitates fluoroscopically directed catheterization of the bile duct most suited for subsequent introduction of a drainage catheter. Random puncture of a bile duct at fine-needle PTC may be disadvantageous for subsequent introduction of a drainage tube.

Immediately after fine-needle PTC the opacified duct system is punctured from the right midaxillary line with a 20-cm mandrin sheathed with a radiopaque polyethylene catheter (OD/ID 1.6/1.0 mm), under biplane fluoroscopic control if available. Penetration of the pleural sinus should be avoided. A peripheral bile duct of the right lobe of the liver should be punctured. This will result in a long intraductal course of the drainage catheter, reducing the risks of catheter dislodgement and intrahepatic vascular lesions. If puncture of a peripheral bile duct is not achieved, a centrally located bile duct should be punctured. When repeated attempts are necessary to achieve puncture the catheter is not completely removed from the liver before renewed insertion of the mandrin, to minimize the trauma to the capsule of the liver. In most cases no more than two to four attempts are necessary. On rare occasions, when only one-plane fluoroscopy is available, up to ten passes of the sheathed mandrin are required before a bile duct suitable for catheterization is entered. During fluoroscopy the puncture of a bile duct can be observed. The tip of the mandrin dislodges the opacified duct slightly before the duct is intentionally crossed by the sheathed mandrin. The mandrin is removed and the catheter is gradually withdrawn until bile is freely aspirated. A guide wire

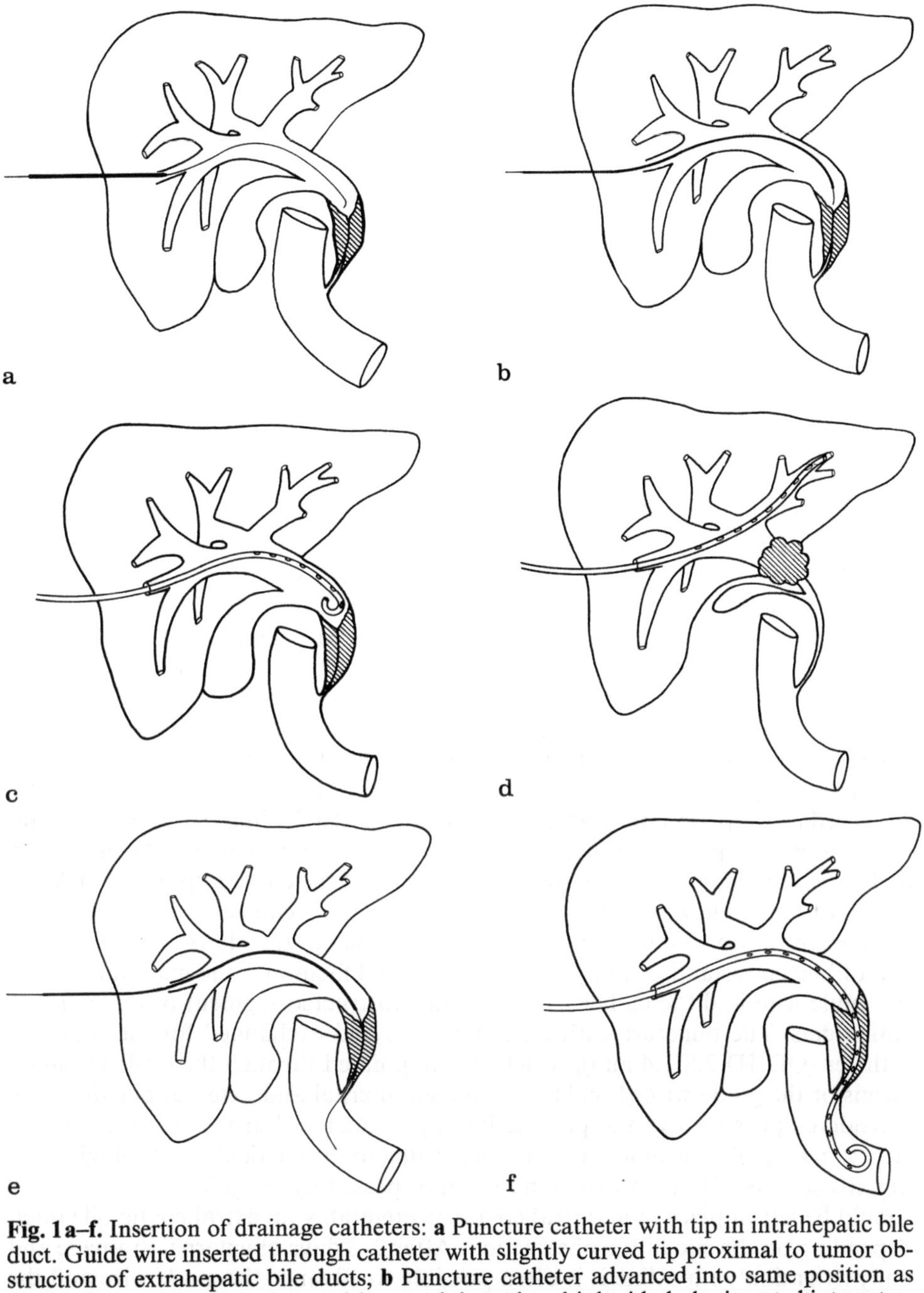


**Fig. 1 a–f.** Insertion of drainage catheters: **a** Puncture catheter with tip in intrahepatic bile duct. Guide wire inserted through catheter with slightly curved tip proximal to tumor obstruction of extrahepatic bile ducts; **b** Puncture catheter advanced into same position as guide wire; **c** Drainage catheter with curved tip and multiple side-holes inserted into extrahepatic bile ducts close to tumor obstruction; **d** Drainage catheter with multiple side-holes inserted into intrahepatic bile ducts. Tip of catheter advanced into bile duct of left liver lobe; **e** Puncture catheter advanced into extrahepatic bile ducts. Guide passed through obstructed bile duct segment with tip in duodenum; **f** Drainage catheter passed through tumor obstruction. Side-holes for internal drainage proximal and distal to site of obstruction

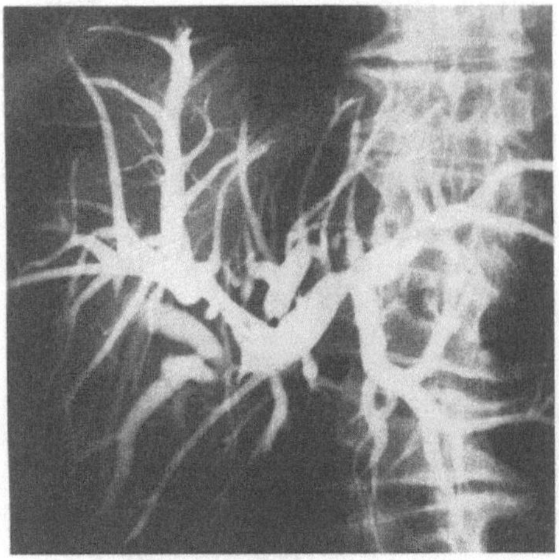

**Fig. 2.** 69-year-old patient with tumor obstruction of common hepatic duct close to confluence of right and left hepatic ducts. Passage of guide wire and catheter through tumor obstruction fails. For external drainage catheter (OD/ID 2.8/1.4 mm) with multiple side-holes inserted into intrahepatic bile ducts. Tip of catheter placed in bile duct of left liver lobe

(0.9 mm) with a soft, slightly curved tip is introduced into the bile duct and manipulated towards the site of the obstruction (Fig. 1 a). The catheter is advanced into the same position (Fig. 1 b). If attempts to pass the biliary duct obstruction with the guide wire are unsuccessful external drainage must be initiated. After removal of the puncture catheter the drainage catheter (OD/ID 2.8/1.4 mm) is inserted by means of the guide wire. The curved tip of the catheter is placed close to the biliary duct obstruction (Fig. 1 c). The drainage catheter is supplied with multiple side-holes. To obtain a stable position of the drainage catheter in patients with obstruction of the proximal segment of the extrahepatic bile ducts the catheter tip should be manipulated into a major intrahepatic bile duct and be advanced as far peripherally as possible (Figs. 1 d and 2). In most cases the guide wire can be manipulated through the stricture of the extrahepatic bile ducts even if obstruction seems complete, by gentle rotation of the curved tip (Fig. 1 e). With the tip of the guide wire in the duodenum the catheter can easily be pushed into the same position. Aspiration of bile from the dilated ductal system reduces the risk of bilivenous and/or bililymphatic reflux and facilitates the manipulation of the guide wire and the catheter through the obstructed segment of the extrahepatic ducts. The puncture catheter is removed and exchanged for the drainage catheter (OD/ID 2.8/1.4 mm), which is manipulated through the obstruction by means of the guide wire (Fig. 1 f). Combined internal and external bile drainage is rendered possible by multiple side-holes proximal and distal to the site of obstruction (Fig. 3). The holes are made according to the particular pathologic findings in each case. If the obstruction cannot be passed by the guide wire, a catheter should be left in place in an intrahepatic or preferably an extrahepatic bile duct, depending on the site of the obstruction. After 2–3 days of external drainage and daily irrigation with saline it is often possible to advance the guide wire and the catheter through the obstruction. Catheter segments with side-holes should not be placed in the parenchyma of the liver, as this may result in a communication between the lumen of the catheter and hepatic vessels, causing hemobilia and/or leakage of possibly infected bile into the blood circulation. In addition to drainage of the bile ducts of the right lobe of the liver, decompression of the bile ducts

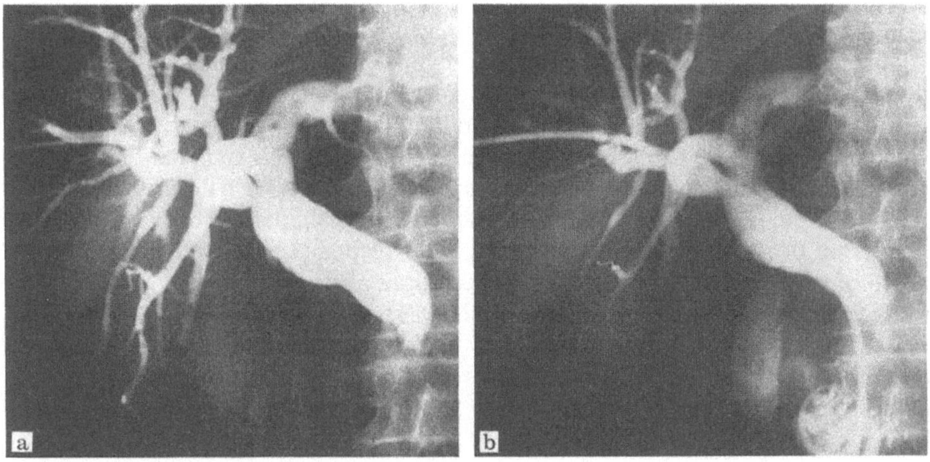

**Fig. 3.** 71-year-old patient with obstructive jaundice due to nonresectable carcinoma of head of pancreas. **a** Following fine-needle PTC a peripheral bile duct of right lobe of liver has been punctured and a catheter (OD/ID 1.6/1.0 mm) advanced into extrahepatic bile ducts. Marked dilatation of intrahepatic bile ducts. Occlusion of common bile duct; **b** For internal and external drainage a catheter (OD/ID 2.8/1.4 mm) has been directed through obstructed segment of common bile duct. Curved tip of catheter in duodenum

of the left lobe can be performed when the obstructive lesion involves the confluence of the hepatic ducts. The bile ducts of the left lobe of the liver are punctured and catheterized from the epigastrium (Jaques et al. 1982; Mueller et al. 1982b).

Regardless of the amount of bile drained externally, the catheter must be flushed with saline at least once a day. The external drain is blocked when the amount of bile drained externally falls below 1 dl/24 h. When a large volume of bile is drained externally appropriate measures have to be taken to restore the loss of water, electrolytes, and bile acids.

If partial catheter dislodgement occurs, the position of the catheter can easily be readjusted with a guide wire, and a more stable position is achieved by pushing it to a position further distal to the obstruction.

## Complications

Percutaneous transhepatic biliary decompression is highly invasive, and a variety of procedure-related complications are on record. The possible damage of the hepatic blood vessels by the puncture needle and the drainage catheter with subsequent formation of pseudoaneurysms, and communications between the hepatic arteries, hepatic and portal veins and the biliary tract has been angiographically demonstrated (Monden et al. 1980; Hoevels and Nilsson 1980; Rosen and Rothberg 1982). Death following intra-abdominal hemorrhage or massive hemobilia has been reported (Hoevels and Nilsson 1980; Mueller et al. 1982a). Slight to moderate bleeding into the biliary tract during the intubation procedure is not rare, and does not indicate a serious complication in the vast majoritiy of cases.

Intraductal blood clots may obstruct the biliary tract for a period of 1–3 days until the clots are dissolved. Fever, chills, and hypotension indicating sepsis may develop during and after the procedure (Mueller et al. 1982a).

Episodes of cholangitis have been reported in patients with long-term transhepatic biliary drainage (Hansson et al. 1979). Cholangitis as a main cause of death in patients with palliative transhepatic biliary drainage has been described (Hansson et al. 1982). Acute pancreatitis secondary to transhepatic biliary intubation for internal drainage with fatal outcome is on record (Luska and Poser 1983). A case of sudden death from multiple pulmonary bile emboli following biliary drainage has been reported (Armellin et al. 1981). Seeding of neoplasm along the tract of a transhepatic drainage tube may occur (Hoevels et al. 1978b; Oleaga et al. 1980).

## References


Ahnlund HO, Morales O (1963) Biliary duct drainage following percutaneous transhepatic cholangiography (in Swedish) Svenska Läkartidningen 60:3685–3691

Armellin GM, Smith RC, Faithful GR (1981) Pulmonary bile emboli following percutaneous cholangiography and biliary drainage. Pathology (Sydney) 13:615–618

Berquist TH, May GR, Johnson CM, Adson MA, Thistle JL (1981) Percutaneous biliary decompression: internal and external drainage in 50 patients. AJR 136:901–906

Burcharth F, Nielbo N (1976) Percutaneous cholangiography with selective catheterization of the common bile duct. AJR 127:409–412

Ferrucci JT Jr, Mueller PR, Harbin WP (1980) Percutaneous transhepatic biliary drainage. Technique, results and applications. Radiology 135:1–13

Hansson JA, Hoevels J, Simert G, Tylén U, Vang J (1979) Clinical aspects of nonsurgical percutaneous transhepatic bile drainage in obstructive lesions of the extrahepatic bile ducts. Ann Surg 189:58–61

Hoevels J, Nilsson U (1980) Intrahepatic vascular lesions following nonsurgical percutaneous transhepatic bile duct intubation. Gastrointest Radiol 5:127–135

Hoevels J, Lunderquist A, Ihse I (1978a) Percutaneous transhepatic intubation of bile ducts for combined internal-external drainage in preoperative and palliative treatment of obstructive jaundice. Gastrointest Radiol 3:23–31

Hoevels J, Lunderquist A, Ihse I (1978b) Percutaneous transhepatic biliary duct intubation for combined internal and external drainage in extrahepatic cholestasis (in German). ROEFO 129:533–550

Jaques PF, Mandell VS, Delaney DJ, Nath PH (1982) Percutaneous transhepatic biliary drainage: advantages of the left-lobe subxiphoid approach. Radiology 145:534–536

Kaude JV, Weidenmier Ch, Agee CF (1969) Decompression of the bile ducts with the percutaneous technique. Radiology 93:69–71

Leger L, Zara et Arvay M (1952) Cholangiography and biliary drainage by means of transhepatic puncture (in French). Presse Méd 42:936–937

Luska G, Poser H (1983) Acute pancreatitis in obstructive jaundice following combined internal and external percutaneous transhepatic bile duct drainage (PTBD). Europ J Radiol 3:112–114

McLean GK, Ring E, Freiman DB (1982) Therapeutic alternatives in the treatment of intrahepatic biliary obstruction. Radiology 145:289–295

Molnar W, Stockum AE (1974) Relief of obstructive jaundice through percutaneous transhepatic catheter – a new therapeutic method. AJR 122:356–367

Monden M, Okamura J, Kobayashi N, Shibata N, Horikawa S, Fujimoto T, Kosaki G, Kuroda C, Uchida H (1980) Hemobilia after percutaneous transhepatic biliary drainage. Arch Surg 115:161–164

Mori K, Misumi A, Sugiyama M, Okabe M, Matsuoka T, Ishii J, Akagi M (1977) Percutaneous transhepatic bile drainage. Ann Surg 185:111–115
Mueller PR, vanSonnenberg E, Ferrucci JT Jr (1982a) Percutaneous biliary drainage: technical and catheter-related problems in 200 procedures. AJR 145:297–302
Mueller PR, Ferrucci JT Jr, vanSonnenberg E, Warshaw AL, Simeone JF, Cronan JJ, Neff CC, Butch RJ (1982b) Obstruction of the left hepatic duct: diagnosis and treatment by selective fine-needle cholangiography and percutaneous biliary drainage. Radiology 145:297–301
Nakayama T, Ikeda A, Okuda K (1978) Percutaneous transhepatic drainage of the biliary tract. Gastroenterology 74:554–559
Ring EJ, Oleaga JA, Freiman DB, Husted JW, Lunderquist A (1978) Therapeutic applications of catheter cholangiography. Radiology 128:333–338
Rosen RJ, Rothberg M (1982) Transhepatic embolization of hepatic artery pseudoaneurysm following biliary drainage. Radiology 145:532–533
Rupp N, Weiss HD, Gain T, Erdt A, Fuessel H (1979) Percutaneous transhepatic biliary duct drainage in obstructive jaundice (in German). ROEFO 130:306–310
Takada T, Hanyu F, Kobayashi S, Uchida Y (1976) Percutaneous transhepatic cholangial drainage: direct approach under fluoroscopic control. J Surg Oncol 8:83–97
Takada T, Uchida Y, Yasuda H, Kobayashi S, Sakakibara N, Hanyu F (1977) Convertion of percutaneous transhepatic cholangiodrainage to internal drainage in obstructive jaundice. Jpn J Surg 7:10–17
Tylén U, Hoevels J, Vang J (1977) Percutaneous transhepatic cholangiography with external drainage of obstructive biliary lesions. Surg Gynecol Obstet 144:13–18

# 5 Complications of Percutaneous Bile Drainage

*J. F. Riemann*

In the last few years, nonsurgical techniques of achieving biliary drainage have developed from virtually unknown methods to efficient, widely accepted procedures (Mori et al. 1977; Burcharth et al. 1979; Köster et al. 1979; Riemann et al. 1981). An invasive therapeutic procedure, external biliary drainage is associated with numerous possibilities for complications (Hoevels et al. 1978; Nakayama et al. 1978; Rupp et al. 1979; Hagenmüller 1982). The aim of the present study was, on the basis of a world-wide survey, to determine the most common complications met with, the way in which they affect the further fate of the individual patient, and the mortality rate of the technique. For this purpose, a questionnaire was designed and sent to 30 centers throughout the world, 18 of which returned the completed questionnaire, so that a representative result may be assumed. The list of participants in this study is outlined in Table 1. The questionnaire was divided up into four parts; in the first part, the indications were specified. The number of procedures carried out for each indication was requested. The success rate was then established, the total number of complications observed, and the average age of the patients involved was recorded. The second part was concerned with the complications. According to a few recent reports and our own experience a differentiation was made between major and minor complications (Ferrucci et

**Table 1.** List of workers participating in the inquiry ($n = 18$)

| | |
|---|---|
| Argentina | A. D. Jorge, Mendoza |
| Brasil | A. J. Ganc, Sao Paulo |
| Denmark | Fl. Burcharth, Copenhagen |
| Germany (West) | R. Köster, B. Swart, Neuss |
| | G. Luska, Hannover |
| | J. F. Riemann, L. Demling, Erlangen |
| | N. Rupp, Munich |
| | L. Safrany, Wilhelmshaven |
| | N. Soehendra, Hamburg |
| Hungary | Z. Döbrönte, V. Varro, Szeged |
| Japan | K. Mori, Kumamoto |
| | T. Nakayama, Kurume |
| | K. Okuda, Chiba |
| South Africa | J. Terblanche, A. Hatfield, Cape Town |
| United Kingdom | P. B. Cotton, London |
| | L. H. Blumgart, G. A. D. McPherson, London |
| United States | J. T. Ferrucci, Boston |
| | E. F. Rosato, Philadelphia |

al. 1980; Riemann et al. 1982). Serious complications were considered to be hemorrhage, hemobilia, bile leakage, biliary peritonitis, sepsis, and development of an abscess, while minor complications were cholangitis without septicemia, pneumothorax, hypotension, hyponatremia, and catheter dislodgement. This questionnaire also requested answers to enquiries as to how the complications were managed, whether they responded to conservative treatment or required emergency surgical treatment, or whether a complication led to the death of the patient. In a third part, information about the indications for the use of a bile duct endoprosthesis inserted percutaneously was requested. The fourth and last sheet of questions dealt with complications and their management.

## Indications for and Complications of Percutaneous Transhepatic Drainage

The total number of biliary drainage procedures evaluated on the above-mentioned basis was 2,471. The main indications, as demonstrated in Table 2, were palliative treatment of malignant bile duct stenoses and, surprisingly frequently, preoperative biliary drainage. These major indications were then followed by the far less frequent benign indications, such as suppurative cholangitis, chronic pancreatitis, bile duct stones, and postoperative biliary duct stenosis. In rare cases, special therapeutic procedures such as litholysis, percutaneous transhepatic bile stone extraction, and the dilatation of strictured bilio-digestive anastomoses were applied. In all, 558 complications were observed; this represents an incidence of 22.6%. Major complications occurred in 15.2% of cases. Of the major complications, the most important were biliary leakage and biliary peritonitis, sepsis, hemobilia and hemorrhage, retroperitoneal or subphrenic abscess, and in rare cases, even renal failure. Among the minor complications, catheter dislodgement, cholangitis without septicemia, difficult-to-control hypotension, hyponatremia and pneumothorax were seen. Table 3 details all the major and minor complications encountered.

**Table 2.** Indication for percutaneous transhepatic biliary drainage ($n = 2,471$)

| | | |
|---|---|---|
| I. *Palliative therapy in malignant bile duct stenoses* | 1,000 | (40.5%) |
| II. *Preoperative biliary drainage* | 1,007 | (40.7%) |
| III. *Benign condition* | | |
| 1. Suppurative cholangitis | 114 | (4.7%) |
| 2. Chronic pancreatitis | 31 | (1.3%) |
| 3. Intrahepatic and/or common bile duct stones | 163 | (6.7%) |
| 4. Postoperative bile duct stricture | 29 | (1.1%) |
| IV. *Special therapeutic procedures* | | |
| 1. Litholysis | 12 | (0.4%) |
| 2. Percutaneous transhepatic gallstone extraction | 6 | (0.2%) |
| 3. Dilatation of strictured bilio-digetive anastomoses | 8 | (0.3%) |
| V. *Two or more catheters* | 101 | (4.1%) |
| | 2,471 | (100.0%) |

**Table 3.** Complications following percutaneous transhepatic biliary drainage ($n = 2{,}471$)

| | | | |
|---|---|---|---|
| Major | | | |
| Bile leakage/biliary peritonitis | | 49 | (2.0%) |
| Sepsis | | 42 | (1.7%) |
| Hemobilia | | 41 | (1.6%) |
| Hemorrhage | | 39 | (1.6%) |
| Retroperitoneal/subphrenic abscess | | 10 | (0.4%) |
| Renal failure | | 2 | (0.1%) |
| | | 183 | (7.4%) |
| Minor | | | |
| Catheter displacement | | 164 | (6.6%) |
| Cholangitis (without septicemia) | | 146 | (5.9%) |
| Hypotension | | 33 | (1.3%) |
| Hyponatremia | | 25 | (1.0%) |
| Pneumothorax | | 7 | (0.3%) |
| | | 375 | (15.2%) |
| | Total | 558 | (22.6%) |

**Table 4.** Management of major complications ($n = 183$) of percutaneous transhepatic biliary drainage ($n = 2{,}471$)

| | Conservative management satisfactory | Emergency surgery necessary | Death rate (drainage-related) |
|---|---|---|---|
| Bile leakage/biliary peritonitis | 26 | 23 | 7 |
| Sepsis | 38 | – | 4 |
| Hemobilia | 34 | 2 | 2 |
| Hemorrhage | 18 | 18 | 8 |
| Retroperitoneal/subphrenic abscess | 18 | 2 | 4 |
| Renal failure | 8 | – | – |
| | 2 | | |
| | 132 (72%) | 45 (24.6%) | 25 (13.7%) |

*Management*

In the case of the major complications, in particular biliary leakage and biliary peritonitis, it was found that it was possible to treat only half of the cases by conservative means, while the other half required emergency surgery (Table 4). Among, these patients, as might be expected, the mortality rate was relatively high. Every case of sepsis responded to conservative therapy, although here, too, four deaths were observed. Hemobilia usually responded to conservative treatment, surgical intervention being needed in only two cases. Two deaths were reported. In the case of hemorrhage, too, the patients could be divided into two halves; one half responded to conservative treatment, while the other required surgery. As expected, here too, the mortality rate with eight deaths, was relatively

**Table 5.** Management of minor complications ($n=375$) of percutaneous transhepatic biliary drainage ($n=2,471$)

| | Conservative management satisfactory | Catheter replacement | Emergency surgery necessary | Death rate (drainage-related) |
|---|---|---|---|---|
| Catheter displacement | 15 | 139 | 4 | 6 |
| Cholangitis (without septicemia) | 64 | 82 | – | 1 |
| Hypotension | 32 | – | – | 1 |
| Hyponatremia | 24 | – | – | 1 |
| Pneumothorax | 6 | – | – | 1 |
| | 141 (37.6%) | 221 (58.9%) | 4 (1%) | 10 (2.5%) |

**Table 6.** Mortality associated with percutaneous transhepatic biliary drainage ($n=2,471$)

| | | |
|---|---|---|
| Deaths due to minor complications | 10 | (0.4%) |
| Deaths due to major complications | 25 | (1.0%) |
| Total deaths | 35 | (1.4%) |

high. Surprisingly, the abscesses that developed, very frequently proved amenable to conservative therapy; in only two cases did surgery have to be performed. However, the mortality rate, with four patients, was relatively high. Renal failure was controlled by conservative measures in every case. Thus it was found that of the 183 reported major complications, 132 (72%) responded to conservative treatment, while in 45 cases (24.6%) surgical intervention proved necessary. The overall mortality rate for the major complications was 25/183, that is 13.7%.

In the treatment of the minor complications (Table 5), a striking feature was that in 15 cases it was possible to deal with catheter dislodgement without the need to replace the catheter; in 139 cases, as expected, the catheter had to be replaced. However, in this connection, too, emergency surgery had to be performed on four occasions. Surprisingly, six deaths were reported for this complication. Cholangitis without septicemia responded to conservative therapeutic measures in 64 cases; in 82 cases the catheter had to be replaced by another. Here, one death was reported. As might be expected, severe hypotension always responded to conservative treatment. Surprisingly, however, here, as also for hyponatremia, one death occurred, three medical treatment instituted obviously not having been adequate. Pneumothorax, which was relatively rarely reported, led to the death of the patient in one case. Thus, of the 375 less serious complications, 144 (37.6%) proved amenable to conservative treatment; in 221 cases (58.9%) the catheter had to be replaced; in 4 cases (1%) emergency surgery was required. The number of deaths was 10, or 2.5%. Considerable importance must thus be attached to the fact that even minor complications can lead to the death of the patient. If the mortality rates are related to the total group (Table 6), we arrive at 10 cases (0.4%) for the minor complications and 25 cases (1%) for the major complications. This corresponds to an overall mortality rate of 1.4%. If this is seen against the background of the severity of the usually underlying clinical picture and the possible complications, this drainage-related mortality rate is quite surprisingly low. No deaths were observed among patients with nonmalignant disease. The complication rate is obviously linked with the experience of the doctor: The center with the lowest number of procedure (n=40) had the highst complication rate (78%), whereas the most experienced team (450 procedures) had only 14% complications.

## Indications for and Complications of Endoprosthesis

The main indications for bile duct endoprostheses introduced percutaneously, a procedure that was carried out in 493 cases, was again the palliative treatment of malignant bile duct stenosis, which accounted for 86.4% of the cases, followed by preoperative biliary drainage in 7.7%, postoperative common bile duct stricture in 2.6%, chronic pancreatitis in 3%, and sclerosing cholangitis in 0.2% (Table 7). The total number of complications observed with this method was 103, or 20.8% (Table 8). Major complications were seen in 47 cases (9.5%) and minor

**Table 7.** Indications for insertion of bile duct endoprosthesis by percutaneous transhepatic approach ($n=493$)

| | | |
|---|---|---|
| I. Palliative therapy in malignant bile duct stenoses | 426 | (86.4%) |
| II. Preoperative biliary drainage | 38 | (7.8%) |
| III. Postsurgical bile duct stricture | 13 | (2.6%) |
| IV. Chronic pancreatitis | 15 | (3.0%) |
| V. Sclerosing cholangitis | 1 | (0.2%) |
| | 493 | (100.0%) |

**Table 8.** Complications of bile duct endoprosthesis inserted by percutaneous transhepatic approach ($n=493$)

| | | |
|---|---|---|
| Major | | |
| Sepsis | 12 | (2.4%) |
| Bile leakage/biliary peritonitis | 11 | (2.2%) |
| Hemorrhage | 11 | (2.2%) |
| Hemobilia | 9 | (1.8%) |
| Retroperitoneal/subphrenic abscess | 4 | (0.9%) |
| | 47 | (9.5%) |
| Minor | | |
| Colangitis (without septicemia) | 20 | (4.1%) |
| Catheter occlusion | 16 | (3.2%) |
| Catheter displacement | 14 | (2.8%) |
| Hypotension | 5 | (1.0%) |
| Pneumothorax | 1 | (0.2%) |
| | 56 | (11.3%) |
| Total | 103 | (20.8%) |

**Table 9.** Management of major complications ($n=47$) of bile duct endoprosthesis inserted by percutaneous transhepatic approach ($n=493$)

| | Conservative management satisfactory | Emergeny surgery necessary | Deaths rate (drainage-related) |
|---|---|---|---|
| Sepsis | 12 | – | – |
| Bile leakage/biliary peritonitis | 6 | 5 | 3 |
| Hemorrhage | 7 | 4 | – |
| Hemobilia | 7 | 1 | 1 |
| Retroperitoneal/subphrenic abscess | 1 | 3 | 1 |
| | 33 (70.2%) | 13 (27.6%) | 5 (10.6%) |

**Table 10.** Management of minor complications ($n=56$) of bile duct endoprosthesis inserted by percutaneous transhepatic approach ($n=493$)

| | Conservative management satisfactory | Emergency surgery necessary | Death rate (drainage-related) |
|---|---|---|---|
| Cholangitis (without septicemia) | 20 | – | – |
| Catheter occlusion | 15 | 1 | – |
| Catheter displacement | 14 | – | 2 |
| Hypotension | 5 | – | – |
| Pneumothorax | 1 | – | – |
| | 55 (98.2%) | 1 (1.8%) | 2 (3.6%) |

**Table 11.** Mortality assosiated with bile duct endoprosthesis inserted by percuteneous transhepatic approach ($n=493$)

| | | |
|---|---|---|
| Deaths due to major complications | 5 | (1.0%) |
| Deaths due to minor complications | 2 | (0.4%) |
| Total deaths | 7 | (1.4%) |

complications in 56 cases (11.3%). The most common major complication was sepsis, followed by biliary leakage and biliary peritonitis, hemorrhage, hemobilia and the development of abscess. The most common minor complication was cholangitis, which was followed by catheter occlusion, catheter dislodgement, hypotension, and pneumothorax.

*Management*

With respect to the therapy of the major complications, sepsis proved to be amenable to conservative treatment in all cases (Table 9). Six cases of biliary leakage responded to conservative measures, in five cases, emergency surgery had to be performed, with three deaths resulting. Seven cases each of bleeding and hemobilia responded to conservative therapy, four other cases of hemorrhage and one of hemobilia having to be treated by emergency surgical intervention; one death was reported. In three cases of retroperitoneal abscess emergency surgery was required, and one death was recorded. This means that of the 47 serious complications, 70.2% responded to conservative treatment, while emergency surgery was required in 27.6%. The mortality rate was 10.6%. More benign complications were, in the main, responsive to conservative measures (Table 10); only in the case of catheter dislodgement were two deaths observed. Of the 56 minor complications, 98.2% were manageable by conservative means, while recourse to emergency surgery was needed in 1.8% of the cases. However, a mortality rate of 3.6% was also seen. Summarizing the overall mortality rate for bile duct endoprosthetic procedures (Table 11) we find that the drainage-related mortality rate for the major complications was 1%, that for the minor complications was 0.4%, and the overall rate was again 1.4%.

## Summary

The data clearly show that percutaneous transhepatic biliary drainage, whether external or in the form of a bile duct endoprothesis, is a therapeutic procedure that is associated with a relatively high risk of complications. Compared with data already published (Burcharth et al. 1979; Ferrucci et al. 1980; Riemann et al. 1982) and the collective data from six centers presented at the Workshop on *Biliary Drainage – Update on Nonsurgical Methods* (Frankfurt, April 1981), the higher overall complication rate may be due to the large number of centers included and presumably may give a more accurate reflection of the complication rate. In both cases, however, the mortality rate is so low that in view of the frequently very poor state of the patient, the use of the procedure is justified.

## References

Burcharth F, Ingemann Jensen L, Olesen K (1979) Endoprosthesis for internal drainage of the biliary tract. Gastroenterology 77:133–137

Ferrucci ST, Mueller PR, Harbin WP (1980) Percutaneous transhepatic biliary drainage. Radiology 135:1–14

Hagenmueller F (1982) Nicht-operative Drainage des Gallengangs. Internist 23:269–272

Hoevels J, Lunderquist A, Ihse J (1978) Percutaneous transhepatic intubation of bile ducts for combined internal-external drainage in preoperative and palliative treatment of obstructive jaundice. Gastrointest Radiol 3:23–28

Köster R, Swart B, Terwort H (1979) Perkutane transhepatische Gallengangsdrainage zur präoperativen und palliativen Behandlung der Gallengangsobstruktion. Radiologe 19:394–404

Nakayama T, Ikeda A, Okuda K (1978) Percutaneous transhepatic drainage of the biliary tract. Gastroenterology 74:554–559

Mori K, Mirumi A, Sugiyama M, Okabe M, Matsucka T, Ishii I, Masanobu A (1977) Percutaneous transhepatic bile drainage. Ann Surg 185:111–116

Riemann JF, Lux G, Roesch W, Beickert-Sterba A (1981) Non-surgical biliary drainage – technique, indications and results. Endoscopy 13:157–161

Riemann JF, Schmack B, Lux G (1982) Perkutane transhepatische Gallenwegsdrainagen. In: Demling L, Riemann JF (eds) Endoskopische Prothetik. Ludwig Heumann & Co, Nürnberg, 20–33

Rupp N, Weiss HD, Vogel G, Gaier Th, Erdt A, Fuestel H (1979) Die perkutane transhepatische Gallengangsdrainage beim Stauungsikterus. ROFO 130:306–313

# 6 Results of Percutaneous External Drainage

*T. Nakayama, H. Saitsu, T. Imamura, M. Sata, S. Yokomizo, M. Yano, T. Isomura, T. Tanaka, and M. Koga*

We have been performing percutaneous transhepatic biliary drainage (PTBD) by various methods since 1965. By 1974, we had established roentgenographically guided PTBD using the movable, J-type guide wire according to Seldinger's method (Nakayama et al. 1978). Simplicity and ease of approach and safety are the primary advantages of this technique. In 1979, we began to apply ultrasonically guided PTBD and the results, with the improved success rates, are reported elsewhere (Tsuchiya and Ebara 1980; Bandai et al. 1980). Table 1 shows the correlation between operative mortality and preoperative total bilirubin value in 412 cases of malignant diseases of the biliary tract (Nakayama et al. 1977). As indicated in Table 1, death frequently occurred when jaundice was bronounced. From 1965 to 1976 PTBD or operative external biliary drainage was applied in the case of expected radical operation. However, a high mortality rate was noted in this period, due to the lack of any means of reducing jaundice in cases when only palliative procedures were expected. Since 1977 PTBD has first been applied in all cases to reduce jaundice, and the operation has been carried out when the bilirubin level has sunk below 5 mg/dl. In contrast, the cases in which it was difficult to reduce jaundice by PTBD were found to have a high mortality. The results indicated that the operative mortality was reduced from 20% to 8% by performing PTBD to reduce jaundice before surgery. Patients with diseases for which PTBD was applied are listed in Table 2. During the 9 years from 1974 to the present, PTBD has been performed in 453 patients, including 346 cases of malignant

**Table 1.** Relation between jaundice and operative mortality [( ) hospital deaths] in patients with malignant biliary obstructions

| Time penod | Serum bilirubin (mg/dl) | | | | | |
|---|---|---|---|---|---|---|
| | ≦1.5 | 1.6 –5 | 5.1 –10 | 10.1 –15 | >15 | Total |
| 1965.1 1976.12 | 45 (2) 4.4% | 17 (1) 5.9% | 17 (3) 17.6% | 30 (6) 20.0% | 115 (33) 28.7% | 224 (45) 20.0% |
| 1977.1 1982.3 | 85 (3) 3.5% | 92 (9) 9.8% | 9 (2) 22.2% | 1 | 1 (1) 100% | 188 (15) 8.0% |
| Total | 130 (5) 3.9% | 109 (10) 9.2% | 26 (5) 19.2% | 31 (6) 19.4% | 116 (34) 29.3% | 412 (60) 14.6% |

**Table 2.** Patients and diseases for which percutaneous transhepatic biliary drainage has been attempted (1974.1–1982.3)

| Diseases | No. of cases |
|---|---|
| Malignant diseases | 346 |
| Bile duct carcinoma | 146 |
| Carcinoma of pancreas | 88 |
| Gallbladder carcinoma | 46 |
| Carcinoma of papilla vater | 30 |
| Recurrent carninoma of stomach | 16 |
| Hepatoma | 9 |
| Cholangioma | 7 |
| Others | 4 |
| Benign diseases | 107 |
| Intrahepatic and common duct stones | 89 |
| Congenital choledochus dilatation | 4 |
| Postoperative strictures of bile duct | 3 |
| Others | 11 |
| Total | 453 |

**Table 3.** Relationship between methods and complications of percutaneous transhepatic biliary drainage

| | Methods of percutaneous transhepatic biliary drainage | |
|---|---|---|
| Complications | Roentgenographically guided drainage | Ultrasonically guided drainage |
| Hemobilia | 5 (1) | 1 |
| Intra-abdominal bleeding | 6 (2) | |
| Hypotension | 20 | 3 |
| Local biliary peritonitis | 3 | 1 |
| Pneumothorax | 1 | |
| Total | 35 (3) | 5 |
| Percent | 35/292 (12%) | 5/161 (3.1%) |

( )death

diseases and 107 cases of benign diseases. Roentgenographically guided PTBD was performed in 292 cases and ultrasonically guided PTBD in 161 cases.

Figure 1 shows a schematic diagram of the roentgenographically guided PTBD procedure we applied during the 6 years from 1974 to 1979. There are two main advantages in this procedure. First, a needle is inserted accurately with determination of the precise position of intrahepatic bile ducts three-dimensionally by means of the frontal and lateral pictures. Second, a drainage tube can also be guided into a target bile duct using a movable J-type guide wire. Figure 2 shows

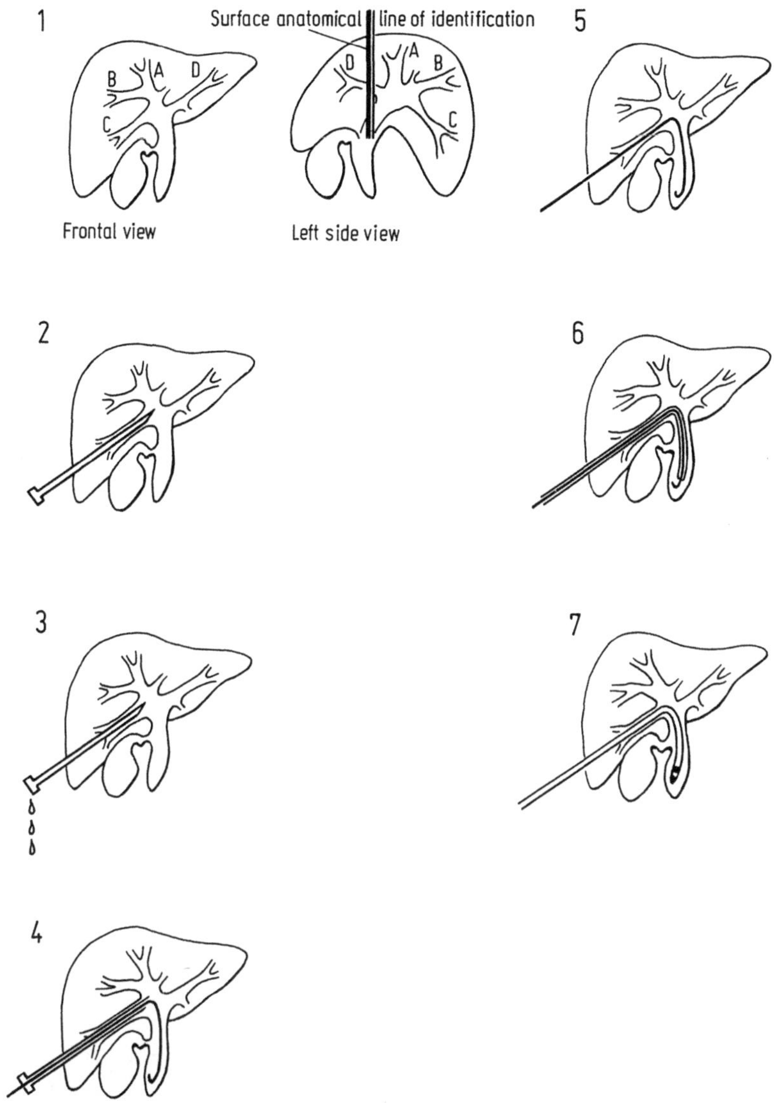


**Fig. 1.** Schematic diagram of the roentgenographically guided PTBD procedure applied by the authors from 1974 to 1979

a schematic diagram of an ultrasonically guided PTBD procedure which has been employed with satisfactory results since 1979. In our experience, drainage with a single-puncture method using a linear-type ultrasonic scanner made it possible to avoid the fall in blood pressure that would otherwise result from the increased bile duct pressure and hemobilia or intra-abdominal bleeding due to accidental insertion of the needle into the intrahepatic vessels (Bandai et al. 1980; Tsuchiya and Ebara 1980). Thus, we could perform drainage more safely and precisely with ul-

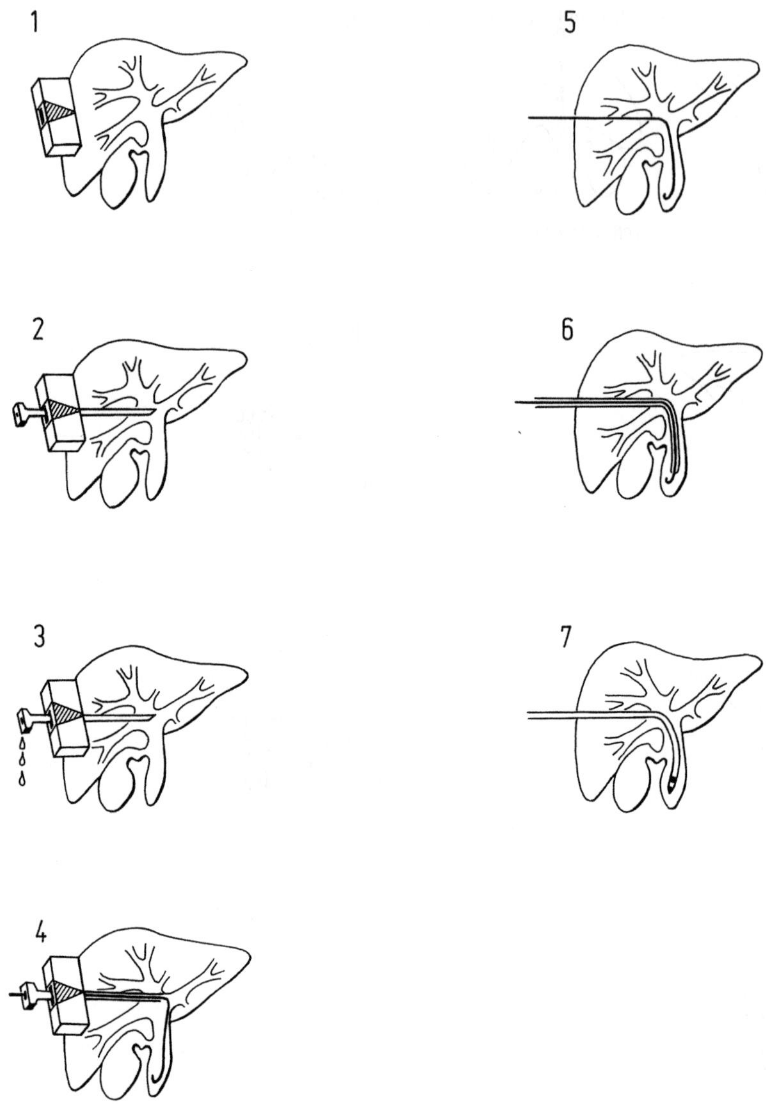


**Fig. 2.** Schematic diagram of an ultrasonically guided PTBD procedure applied by the authors since 1979

trasonically guided PTBD. In most cases, we inserted the drainage tube into the right posterosuperior duct from the right intracostal region (36%) or into the left lateroinferior duct from the epigastrium (23%). Figure 3a shows some instances of ultrasonically guided PTBD.

The success rate of roentgenographically guided PTBD was approximately 98% and a similar result was obtained with our ultrasonically guided PTBD. Table 3 describes the details of complications and mortality following PTBD.

**Fig. 3.** Some examples of ultrasonically guided PTBD. intracostal scanning reveals dilatation of the intrahepatic duct

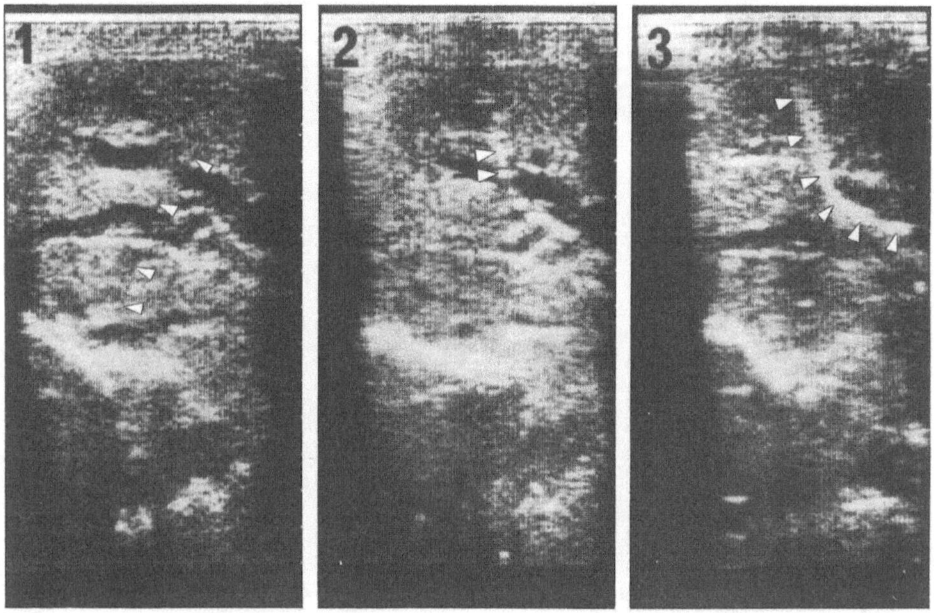


**Fig. 3a.** Puncture of the middle hepatic vein (*left, arrows*) must be carefully avoided. The bile duct is punctured (*middle, arrows* indicate needlee tip): a guide wire is used (*right, arrows*)

Complications were seen in 40 cases among 453, and only 3 patients died of hemobilia or intra-abdominal bleeding. In 292 cases of roentgenographically guided drainage, varying degrees of hemobilia were found in 5 cases, intra-abdominal bleeding in 6 cases, hypotension in 20 cases, local biliary peritonitis in 3 cases, and pneumothorax in 1 case.

However, in 161 cases of ultrasonically guided drainage, hemobilia occurred in 1 case, hypotension in 3 cases, and local biliary peritonitis in 1 case; that is to say complications arose in 5 cases. Additional complications were cholangitis and catheter dislodgement, which were not regarded as direct complications of PTBD. As to cholangitis, our established criteria for diagnosis are remittent fever (over 38 °C), leukocytosis (over 10,000/mm$^3$), and positive bile culture occurring simultaneously.

Cholangitis was seen in 36 (7.9%) of 453 cases and the prognosis was found to be poor in the cases when the agonal stage had been reached. Catheter dislodgement was experienced in 38 cases. In most of these, the postoperative course was uneventful after PTBD had been successfully repeated.

## Summary

Ultrasonically guided drainage seems to prevent hypotension due to increased intrabile duct pressure and bleeding caused by accidental puncture of intrahepatic

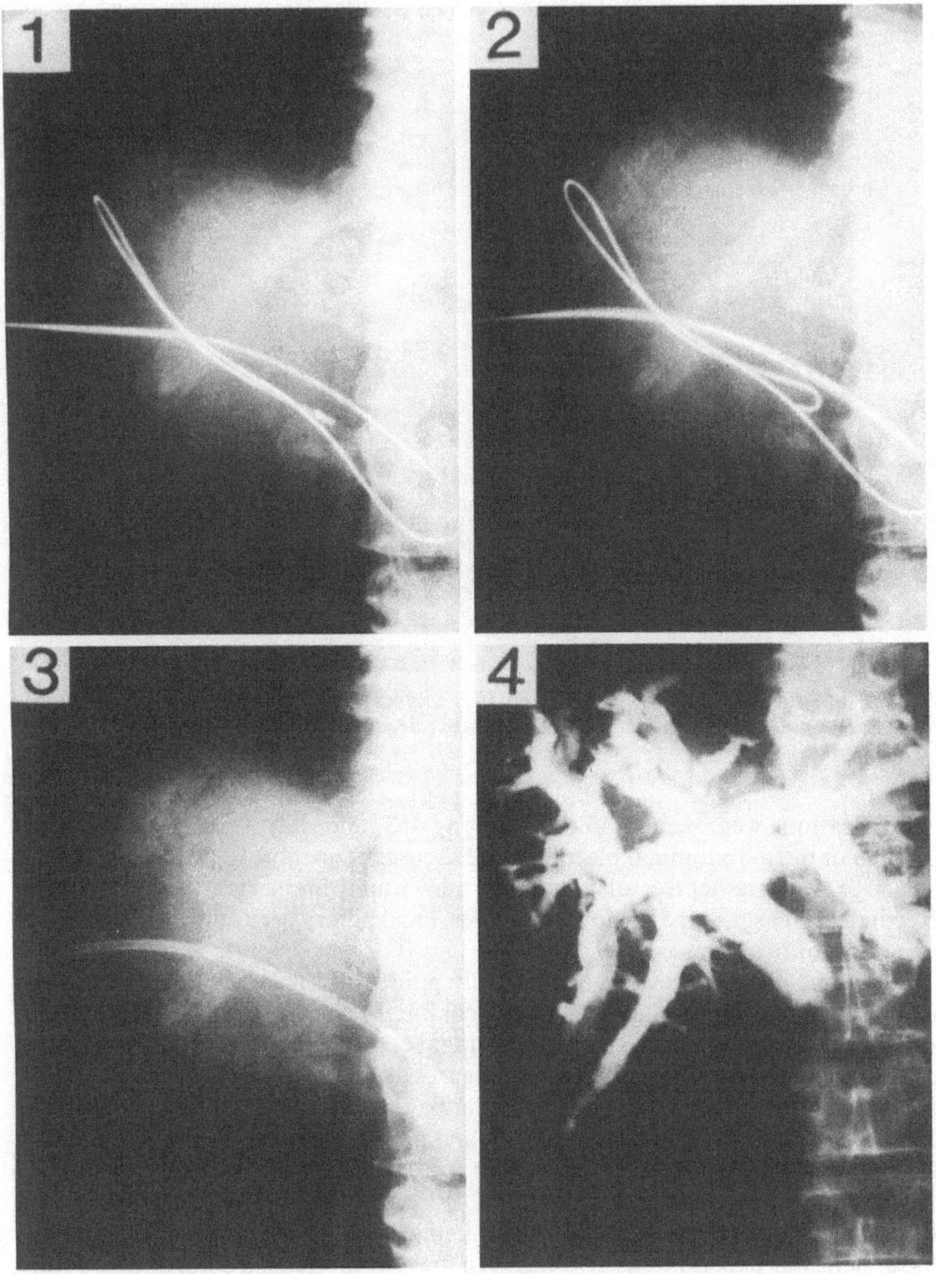


**Fig. 3b.** Cholangiography taken after insertion of the drainage tube with the guide wire with roentgenographic monitoring in a patient with carcinoma of the pancreas

vessels. We have not experienced any mortality with ultrasonically guided PTBD, and the drainage has been performed more safely than when roentgenographically guided.

## References

Bandai Y, Itoh T et al. (1980) Ultrasonically guided percutaneous transhepatic biliary drainage – safer and easier method. J Clin Surg 35:1415–1418

Nakayama T, Muraishi N et al. (1977) Problem point of the surgical treatment for malignant obstructive jaundice. Jpn J Gastroenterol Surg 10:708–714

Nakayama T, Ikeda A et al. (1978) Percutaneous transhepatic drainage of the biliary tract. Gastroenterology 74:554

Tsuchiya Y, Ebara M (1980) A new method for percutaneous transhepatic bile drainage – ultrasonically guided technique. J Clin Surg 35:1409–1413

# 7 Results of Percutaneous Internal-External Drainage

*J. Hoevels and A. Lunderquist*

Transhepatic biliary drainage, in the vast majority of cases, is performed in patients with malignant obstruction of the extrahepatic bile ducts. As an alternative to surgical decompression as a first step in a two-stage procedure, decrease of cholestasis can be achieved by temporary preoperative nonsurgical percutaneous transhepatic catheterization of the bile ducts. A decrease of operative morbidity and mortality secondary to preoperative transhepatic bile duct decompression in patients with extrahepatic cholestasis has been reported (Takada et al. 1976; Nakayama et al. 1978; Denning et al. 1981). Other authors observed no significant difference in postoperative complications and mortality between patients treated with preoperative transhepatic bile drainage and jaundiced patients operated on without prior drainage (Hatfield et al. 1982).

The age and general condition of the jaundiced patient and/or the site of the tumor may preclude operative bile duct decompression. Relief of biliary obstruction by nonsurgical procedures should therefore be considered as an alternative palliative therapy. When the diagnostic workup has shown a cytologically verified malignant bile duct obstruction, patients who may be suitable for permanent palliative nonsurgical biliary duct drainage via a transhepatic catheter include those with: (1) a prohibitively high operative risk; (2) a tumor which is nonresectable as demonstrated by ultrasonography, computed tomography, and angiography; (3) metastases to the liver and/or to distant organs; (4) a metastatic tumor obstructing the extrahepatic bile ducts; and (5) a primary bile duct tumor involving the confluence of the hepatic ducts and the intrahepatic biliary radicles.

In patients undergoing preoperative decompression external drainage as a short-term solution for extrahepatic biliary obstruction is the optimal procedure if internal drainage fails. For palliative treatment it is more advantageous to achieve combined internal and external drainage via a catheter (Fig. 1 a, b). The catheter rests in a more stable position and the depletion of water, bile acids and electrolytes is less pronounced than with external drainage. When the internal bile flow is not impeded, the volume of bile drained externally via the catheter ranges between approximately 1 and 2 dl/24 h. The catheter should be changed after 2–3 months to avoid drainage malfunction secondary to incrustation and sludge within the tube. Increasing external bile flow indicates malfunction of the internal limb of the catheter distal to the biliary duct obstruction. Forced flushing with 10–20 ml saline or passage of a guide wire to clean the catheter may restore internal bile drainage. If this fails it is advisable to replace the drainage catheter by a new one using the guide wire technique. Passage of a catheter through the lesion obstructing the external bile ducts is possible in approximately 70%–80% of

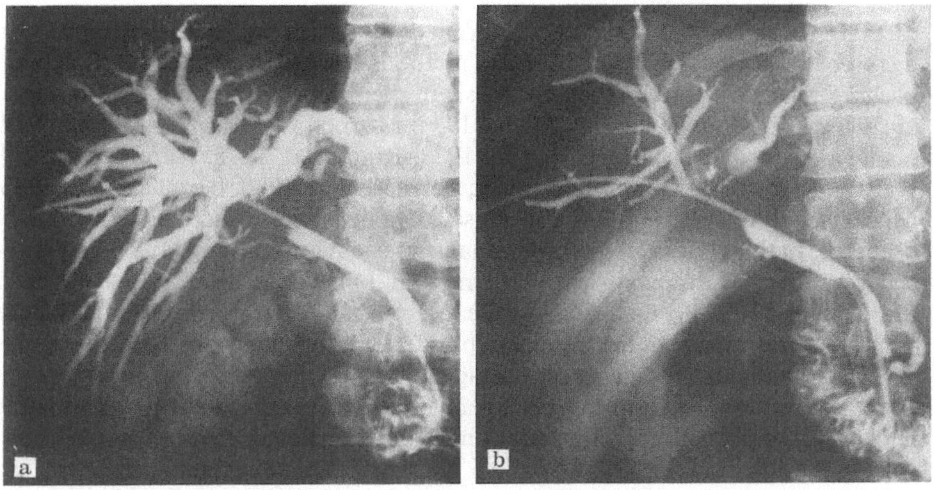

**Fig. 1.** A 44-year-old patient with obstruction of common hepatic duct secondary to metastases from gastric carcinoma. Gastrectomy performed 1 year previously. **a** Drainage catheter (OD/ID 2.8/1.4 mm) manipulated through occluded segment of common hepatic duct. Curved tip of catheter in duodenum. Dilatation of intrahepatic bile ducts. **b** Marked decrease of biliary duct dilatation after 4 days of internal and external drainage.

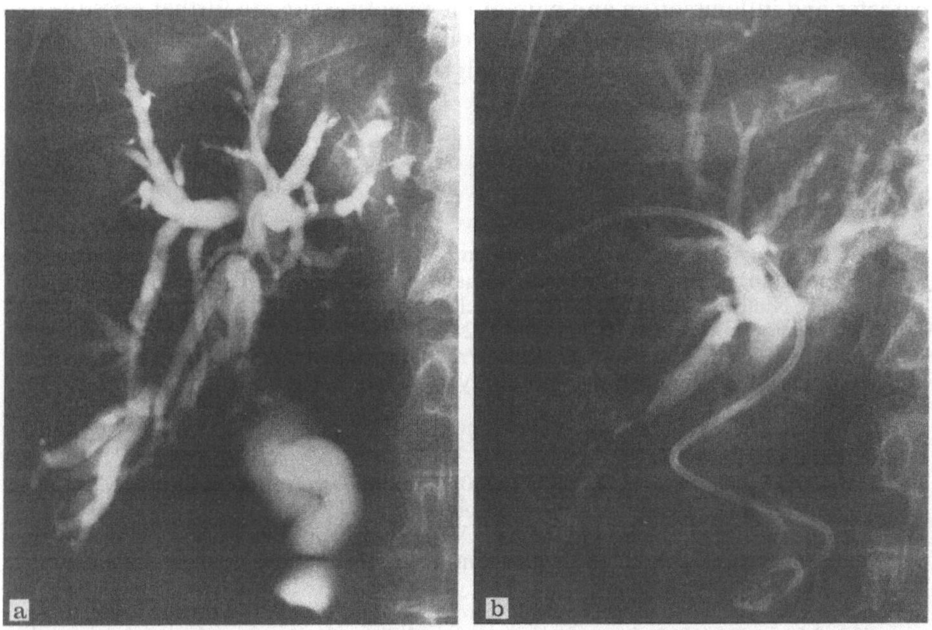

**Fig. 2.** A 71-year-old patient with obstructive jaundice secondary to nonresectable carcinoma of head of pancreas. **a** Fine-needle PTC demonstrates occlusion of common bile duct and dilatation of intrahepatic and extrahepatic bile ducts. **b** Attempts to pass the biliary duct obstruction with catheter for internal-external drainage failed. For external drainage catheter was advanced into extrahepatic bile ducts. Tip of catheter adjacent to tumor occluding common bile duct

cases. In the remainder of patients external drainage for palliative decompression has to be performed (Fig. 2a, b). Both methods have proved effective in accomplishing relief of extrahepatic cholestasis in the majority of patients (Takada et al. 1976, 1977; Burcharth and Nielbo 1976; Mori et al. 1977; Tylén et al. 1977; Nakayama et al. 1978; Hoevels et al. 1978; Ring et al. 1978; Rupp et al. 1979; Hansson et al. 1979; Dooley et al. 1979; Ferrucci et al. 1980; Berquist et al. 1981). Mueller et al. (1982) analyzed 200 consecutive instances of percutaneous biliary drainage. In this series, successful drainage was achieved in 188 (94%) of 200 procedures. Internal drainage was performed in 144 (72%) and external catheter drainage in 44 (22%) instances. McLean et al. (1982) performed percutaneous transhepatic drainage in the treatment of intrahepatic biliary obstruction secondary to cholangiocarcinoma or sclerosing cholangitis. Percutaneous biliary drainage has been advocated in the management of biliary sepsis due to suppurative cholangitis or postsurgical complications (Nakayama et al. 1978; Mason and Irving 1981; Kadir et al. 1982).

There are, however, some shortcomings involved in these methods, especially with regard to long-term palliative treatment. The drainage may be interfered with by spontaneous catheter dislodgement (Hoevels et al. 1978; Ferrucci et al. 1980) or infection of the biliary duct system through the external catheter (Hansson et al. 1979).

External leakage of ascitic fluid or bile around the percutaneous transhepatic catheter and inflammation and pain at the puncture site are further possible disadvantages of the procedure. These obvious disadvantages are avoidable when internal biliary drainage is achieved through a transhepatically inserted endoprosthesis.

## References


Berquist TH, May GR, Johnson CM, Adson MA, Thistle JL (1981) Percutaneous biliary decompression: internal and external drainage in 50 patients. AJR 136:901–906

Burcharth F, Nielbo N (1976) Percutaneous cholangiography with selective catheterization of the common bile duct. AJR 127:409–412

Denning DA, Ellison EC, Carey LC (1981) Preoperative percutaneous transhepatic biliary decompression lowers operative morbidity in patients with obstructive jaundice. Am J Surg 141:61–64

Dooley JS, Dick R, Olney J, Sherlock S (1979) Non-surgical treatment of biliary obstruction. Lancet II:1040–1043

Ferrucci JT Jr, Mueller PR, Harbin WP (1980) Percutaneous transhepatic biliary drainage. Technique, results and applications. Radiology 135:1–13

Hansson JA, Hoevels J, Simert G, Tylén U, Vang J (1979) Clinical aspects of nonsurgical percutaneous transhepatic bile drainage in obstructive lesions of the extrahepatic bile ducts. Ann Surg 189:58–61

Hatfield ARW, Tobias R, Terblanche J, Girdwood AH, Fataar S, Harries-Jones R, Kernoff L, Marks IN (1982) Preoperative external biliary drainage in obstructive jaundice. Lancet II:896–899

Hoevels J, Lunderquist A, Ihse I (1978) Percutaneous transhepatic intubation of bile ducts for combined internal-external drainage in preoperative and palliative treatment of obstructive jaundice, Gastrointest Radiol 3:23–31

Kadir S, Baassiri A, Barth KH, Kaufman SL, Cameron JL, White RI Jr (1982) Percutaneous biliary drainage in the management of biliary sepsis. AJR 138:25–29

McLean GK, Ring E, Freiman DB (1982) Therapeutic alternatives in the treatment of intrahepatic biliary obstruction. Radiology 145:289–295
Mason RR, Irving JD (1981) Resolution of multiple abscesses following percutaneous transhepatic biliary drainage. Br J Radiol 54:391–393
Mori K, Misumi A, Sugiyama M, Okabe M, Matsuoka T, Ishii J, Akagi M (1977) Percutaneous transhepatic bile drainage. Ann Surg 185:111–115
Mueller PR, vanSonnenberg E, Ferrucci JT Jr (1982) Percutaneous biliary drainage: technical and catheter-related problems in 200 procedures. AJR 138:17–23
Nakayama T, Ikeda A, Okuda K (1978) Percutaneous transhepatic drainage of the biliary tract. Gastroenterology 74:554–559
Ring EJ, Oleaga JA, Freiman DB, Husted JW, Lunderquist A (1978) Therapeutic applications of catheter cholangiography. Radiology 128:333–338
Rupp N, Weiss HD, Vogel G, Gain T, Erdt A, Fuessel H (1979) Percutaneous transhepatic biliary duct drainage in obstructive jaundice (in german) ROEFO 130:306–310
Takada T, Hanyu F, Kobayashi S, Uchida Y (1976) Percutaneous transhepatic cholangial drainage: direct approach under fluoroscopic control. J Surg Oncol 8:83–97
Takada T, Uchida Y, Yasuda H, Kobayashi S, Sakakibara N, Hanyu F (1977) Conversion of percutaneous transhepatic cholangiodrainage to internal drainage in obstructive jaundice. Jpn J Surg 7:10–17
Tylén U, Hoevels J, Vang J (1977) Percutaneous transhepatic cholangiography with external drainage of obstructive biliary lesions. Surg Gynecol Obstet 144:13–18

# 8 Results of the Percutaneous Implantation of Endoprostheses

*F. Burcharth*

Nonoperative biliary drainage effected by leaving the cannula or catheter in a bile duct after percutaneous transhepatic cholangiography was first reported some 20 years ago (Glenn et al. 1962). No attempt was made to position the catheter, because surgery was scheduled fo follow shortly after the diagnostic procedure. Some years later, several groups documented the feasibility of introducing catheters transhepatically into an obstructed biliary tree and through strictures, and the safety and therapeutic potential of short- or long-term transhepatic external and/or internal bile drainage were reported (Molnar and Stockum 1974; Burcharth et al. 1976, 1977; Takada et al. 1976; Mori et al. 1977; Hoevels et al. 1978; Nakayama et al. 1978; Ring et al. 1978; Ferrucci et al. 1980).

Internal drainage without an external catheter, by transhepatic insertion of an endoprosthesis, has been used since 1972 (Burcharth 1978), and a number of authors have since described the use of this method (Pereiras et al. 1978; Burcharth et al. 1979, 1981; Hoevels and Ihse 1979; Dooley et al. 1979, 1981; Rupp and Weiss 1980). Compared with external bile drainage, this procedure does not deplete patients of bile, water, and electrolytes, and it is not as uncomfortable and depressing for the patient.

This paper describes the transhepatic technique of inserting endoprostheses through biliary strictures, and gives a multi-institutional survey of the results.

## Patients and Methods

The data were collected in 9 hospitals in Western Europe and the United States (listed below). Between December 1972 and April 1982 insertion of a biliary endoprosthesis was attempted in 455 patients, the majority within the last 4 years. A median of 25 patients have been treated by this approach in each hospital, with a range of 4–204 patients. The median age of the patients treated for malignant conditions was 70 years, with a range of 16–94 years.

**Table 1.** Diseases for which insertion of endoprosthesis was attempted ($n=455$)

| | | | |
|---|---|---|---|
| Malignant stenosis | | Benign stenosis | |
| Intrahepatic bile duct stenosis (including hilar obstructions) | 133 | Postoperative bile duct stricture | 15 |
| Extrahepatic bile duct stenosis (excluding periampullary tumors) | 137 | Chronic pancreatitis | 13 |
| Periampullary stenosis (including pancreatic cancer) | 146 | Sclerosing cholangitis | 4 |
| | | Other conditions (including suppurative cholangitis) | 7 |
| Total | 416 (91%) | | 39 (9%) |

**Table 2.** Number of patients with transhepatic endoprosthesis for permanent or temporary internal biliary drainage

| No. of cases | Success rate | Palliative (permanent) treatment | Preoperative (temporary) drainage | Two or more endoprosthesis |
|---|---|---|---|---|
| 455 | 402 (88%) | 353 (88%) | 49 (12%) | 44 (10%) |

Biliary obstruction was caused by a malignant lesion in 416 patients (91%) (Table 1). The lesions were equally distributed in the biliary tract. Most of the 39 benign lesions were due to postoperative stricture and chronic pancreatitis (Table 1).

In 49 patients (12%) elective surgery had been planned, and the endoprosthesis was inserted to provide preoperative internal drainage (Table 2).

The *indications* for insertion of an endoprosthesis were: *Temporary drainage prior to surgery* for obstructing common duct stones, benign stenoses or tumors; *permanent drainage in inoperable lesions,* either benign or malignant; and a *prohibitively high operative risk.*

## *Technique*

Before transhepatic catheterization of the bile ducts is attempted, dilated intrahepatic ducts should be demonstrated either by ultrasonic examination or by fine-needle cholangiography. Severe coagulopathies contraindicate transhepatic catheterization. If obstruction is demonstrated by fine-needle cholangiography, catheterization and drainage must be established immediately to avoid cholangitis.

The patient is prepared, fasted, and premedicated as for routine transhepatic cholangiography. The diagnostic cholangiogram is performed with a fine needle (0.7 mm) under local anesthesia. The lateral approach through the 7th or 8th intercostal space in the midaxillary line is used. A sheathed needle (1.0–1.4 mm) is then passed into the bile duct and a further cholangiogram is performed (Burcharth and Nielbo 1976; Burcharth et al. 1977). A flexible guide wire (0.9 mm) with a slightly curved tip is passed under fluoroscopic control into the hepatic or common bile duct, and advanced to the obstruction. The catheter is threaded over the guide wire, which is subsequently removed (Fig. 1). When a catheter is placed in the intrahepatic bile ducts just above the obstruction, the guide wire tip can usually be directed under fluoroscopic control into the entrance of the lumen of the stricture. The critical maneuver in the procedure is the passage of the guide wire through the obstruction. A bend near the tip of the guide wire and manipulation by rotation is often essential for successful insertion (Fig. 2). If the guide wire cannot be advanced past the obstruction, external drainage is established for 2–4 days, after which a further attempt is made. There is usually a reduction in the edematous swelling of the duct wall above the obstruction, so that cannulation of the stricture is then possible.

Several designs of endoprostheses are available commercially. Most are 6–15 cm long radiopaque polythylene tubes with multiple side holes, and diameters from 2.0 to 4.0 mm. Some are straight, smooth, and flexible, while others are rigid with a preformed shape.

The insertion is performed by means of an introducer of the same diameter as the endoprosthesis. The introducer is threaded over the guide wire, which has been passed through the obstruction. The largest size of introducer which can be passed through the obstruction is found. The introducer is then removed, and the corresponding size of endoprosthesis is pushed through the obstruction with the introducer. The endoprosthesis is placed with the distal end below the obstruction, sometimes in the duodenum, and the proximal end in an intrahepatic duct above the obstruction (Fig. 3). Protrusion of the endoprosthesis through the papilla may be important, particularly in patients with benign strictures, as this offers the possibility of endoscopic removal. The introducers or a standard external drainage catheter is left in the punctured intrahepatic or hepatic duct to provide temporary external drainage and to prevent bleeding and bile leakage from the punc-

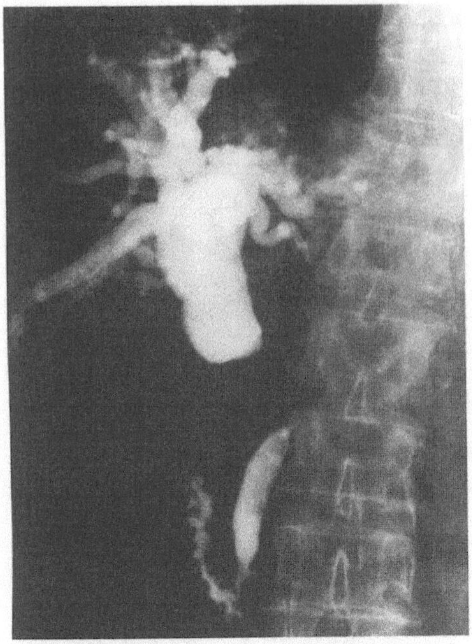

**Fig. 1.** Percutaneous transhepatic cholangiography demonstrating a malignant stenosis in the common bile duct

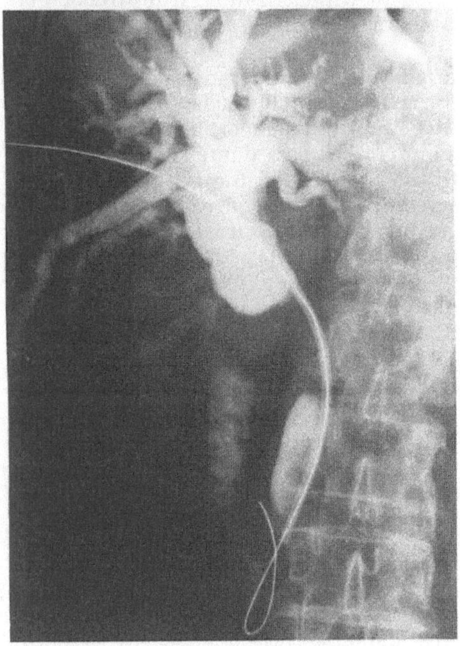

**Fig. 2.** Flexible guide wire manipulated through the stricture

ture site. Cholangiograms can be performed through this catheter to check the function of the endoprosthesis. The external catheter is clamped after 3–4 days when the external bile flow has decreased, and then it is withdrawn stepwise over a 12-h period. Routine antibiotic cover is not given. Prophylactic antibiotics are only used if calculi are suspected or if there is an anastomosis between biliary system and bowel, when the risk of biliary infection is high.

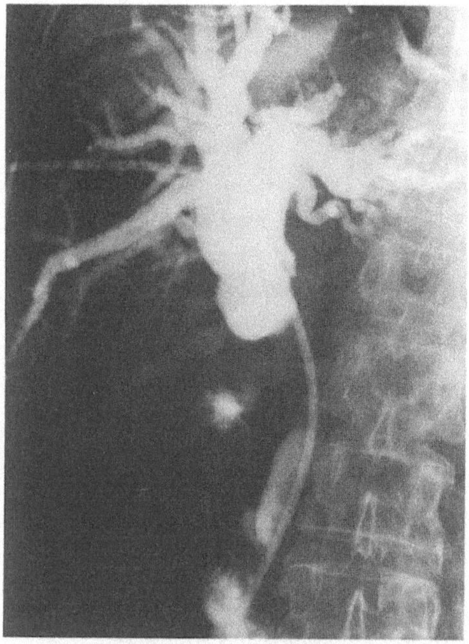

**Fig. 3.** Endoprosthesis introduced and passed through the stricture. The introducer left in an intrahepatic duct for temporary external drainage

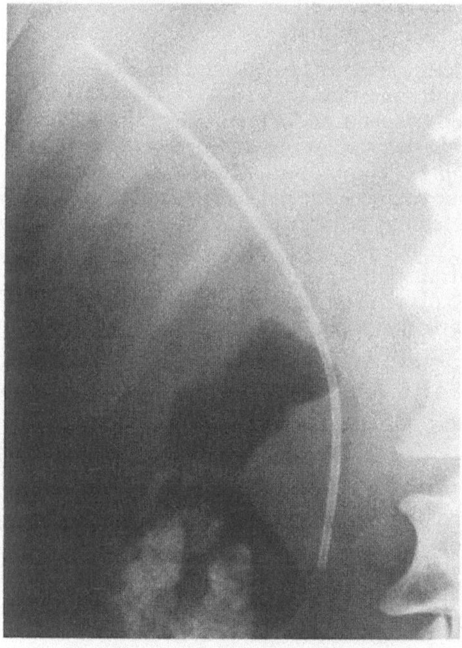

**Fig. 4.** Plain abdominal x-ray after withdrawal of the external drain, showing the endoprosthesis in the correct position

When insertion of the large, rigid type of endoprosthesis with preformed shape is preferred, dilatation of the stricture with a dilatation catheter is essential before insertion of the endoprosthesis. To facilitate insertion a stiff guide wire with a flexible distal end is helpful.

Nearly all endoprostheses can be inserted under local anesthesia with intravenous sedation and analgesia at the time of the procedure. The local anesthetic agent should not

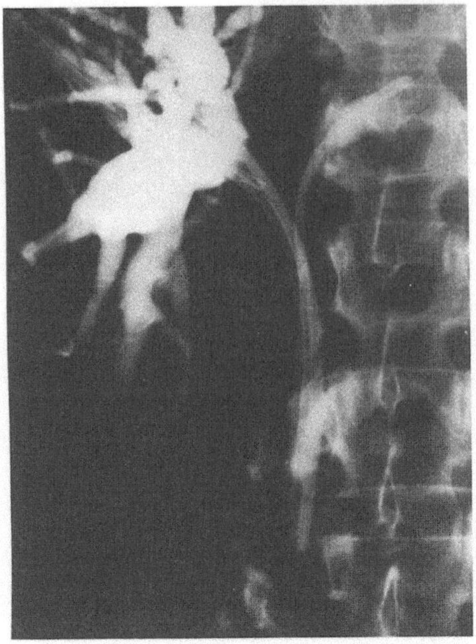

**Fig. 5.** Three endoprostheses inserted, one from each duct system, in a patient with sclerosing cholangitis and multiple stenoses

only be injected in the intercostal space at the puncture site, but also around the intercostal nerve to provide adequate and sufficiently long-lasting anesthesia.

The position of the endoprosthesis is controlled by plain abdominal x-rays (Fig. 4); its function may be assessed by serial plasma bilirubin determinations and if necessary duodenoscopy or fine-needle cholangiography. Flushing of the endoprosthesis is not possible, but a non-functioning endoprosthesis can be removed with the aid of the duodenoscope and a new one inserted, or additional endoprostheses may be inserted. In patients with multiple intrahepatic strictures drainage of more than one segment of the liver can be achieved by insertion of endoprostheses from different intrahepatic bile ducts (Fig. 5).

An anterior subcostal approach may be used to place an endoprosthesis through the left hepatic duct (Fig. 5) (Takada et al. 1976; Burcharth 1982). In such cases, preliminary ultrasonic localization of the dilated left hepatic duct is often a useful maneuver.

## Results

Insertion of an endoprosthesis was successful in 402 patients (88%) (Table 2); and 44 patients (10%) had more than one endoprosthesis inserted.

**Table 3.** Immediate complications of insertion of endoprosthesis in 455 patients

| | *n* | % |
|---|---|---|
| Bile leakage | 16 | 3.5 |
| Intra-abdominal bleeding | 8 | 1.8 |
| Pneumothorax | 1 | 0.2 |
| Total | 25 | 5.5 |

**Table 4.** Late complications of permanent endoprostheses in 402 patients

| | $n$ | % |
|---|---|---|
| Cholangitis (with septicemia) | 23 | 5.7 |
| Perihepatic abscess | 9 | 2.2 |
| Other[a] | 17 | 4.2 |
| Total | 49 | 12.1 |
| Dislodgment of endoprosthesis | 14 | 3.5 |

[a] Perforations of duodenum, 2; hemobilia, 1; portal vein thrombosis, 1

**Table 5.** Effect of endoprosthesis on jaundice in 283 patients with permanent endoprosthesis for malignant stenosis

| Effect on jaundice | $n$ | % |
|---|---|---|
| Disappeared | 188 | 66 |
| Moderate effect | 48 | 17 |
| No effect | 47 | 17 |

Twenty-five patients (5.5%) had *immediate complications* to the insertion, predominantly bile leakage and hemorrhage (Table 3). The most common *late complication* was cholangitis, which occurred in 23 patients (6%) (Table 4). Nine patients had subphrenic or subhepatic abscesses. In 14 patients (3.5%) the endoprosthesis became dislodged, most frequently into duodenum. Seventeen (23%) of the complications demanded surgical intervention. Seven patients (1.5%) died due to bile leakage and bile peritonitis and/or cholangitis with septicemia.

Long-term follow-up was possible in 283 of the 329 patients (86%) with permanent endoprostheses for malignant stenosis. The plasma bilirubin concentration decreased to normal or subclinical levels in 66% (Table 5). In 17% the decrease was moderate, and in 17% the bilirubin level showed only a slight decrease, remained unchanged, or rose. The median survival was 3.2 months, with a range of less than 1 month to 35 months. Twenty-seven of these patients are still alive. The mean survival of the patients who died was 4 months. Survival was somewhat longer for those patients who survived the first month and who had marked reduction of the plasma bilirubin concentration. Survival was related neither to the type of malignant disease nor to its localization.

## Discussion

Surgical therapy remains the primary treatment in patients with resectable lesions, because of the possibility of cure, but 80%–90% of malignant biliary obstructions are nonresectable (Hermann and Cooperman 1979). Operative drainage in patients with nonpancreatic malignant obstructions has a mortality of approximately 20%, increasing to 30% in pancreatic cancer (Feduska et al. 1971; Burcharth et al. 1981). If widespread metastases are present, the mortality rises further (Feduska et al. 1971). In patients with hilar stricture, including those with metastatic disease at the porta hepatis, it is often technically impossible to construct any anastomosis. The percutaneous transhepatic insertion of an endoprosthesis through the stricture at the time of cholangiography is an attractive alternative to surgery, and allows palliation for some patients with advanced cancer which would otherwise be impossible to achieve.

Previously the only management available for patients with benign strictures was surgical. Many patients with postoperative strictures have had multiple operations, and surgical repair becomes increasingly difficult. Relief of benign strictures with an endoprosthesis should be considered (Burcharth and Pedersen 1981; Burcharth et al. 1981; Dooley et al. 1981).

Surgery in patients with marked obstructive jaundice is associated with an increased risk of postoperative complications (Feduska et al. 1971; Braasch and Gray 1977; Nakayama et al. 1978). Transhepatic drainage, including endoprothesis insertion has been used preoperatively to reduce the risk (Nakayama et al. 1978; Denning et al. 1981), but controlled trials are necessary to evaluate the effect of such treatment on operative mortality and morbidity. Another indication for temporary transhepatic drainage has been the emergency management of acute suppurative cholangitis (Takada et al. 1976; Dooley et al. 1979; Ferrucci et al. 1980).

Relief of cholestasis by means of the endoprosthesis was not achieved in every patient in this study. Many patients with malignant disease died soon after the procedure due to their poor clinical state and underlying pathology, and in these patients the effect of drainage on jaundice could not be evaluated. The relief of jaundice in 66% of the patients with permanent endoprostheses is similar to that achieved by external/internal transhepatic drainage (Burcharth 1982), without the disadvantages of a transhepatic drainage catheter. The median survival time of 3.2 months was rather short. In patients with nonresectable periampullary tumors, the results after bypass surgery have been compared with treatment by transhepatic endoprosthesis (Burcharth et al. 1981). Assessed by the effect on jaundice and survival time, nonsurgical biliary drainage by an endoprosthesis was as effective as a surgical anastomosis.

The immediate complications of insertion of an endoprosthesis were essentially the same as those seen after diagnostic transhepatic cholangiography, and the frequency was only slightly higher. To avoid bile leakage and bleeding, the biliary system must always be entered intrahepatically, so that the puncture is sealed by liver tissue, and a drainage catheter must be left for temporary external drainage of bile. A surgical team should be informed before endoprosthesis insertion is performed. The external catheter is only removed when internal drainage of bile is proven.

The most common and serious late complication of long-term biliary drainage is cholangitis. The frequency of severe cholangitis is about 20% with transhepatic external/internal drainage catheters (Hoevels et al. 1978; Ferrucci et al. 1980; Burcharth 1982). Cholangitis with septicemia occurred is only about 6% of the patients with an endoprosthesis, even though many of the endoprostheses protruded through the papilla and prophylactic antibiotics were given only in a minority of patients. The external part of the catheter is probably responsible for the high frequency of cholangitis with transhepatic drainage catheters.

Other complications occurred infrequently. Hemobilia is rather uncommon (Moden et al. 1980). Even though arteriovenous shunts have been shown to occur after transhepatic catheterization procedures, they probably have no clinical implications (Okuda et al. 1978). Two endoprostheses caused perforation of the duodenum shortly after the insertion. The perforations may have been caused by the insertion procedure. No perforations of the bile ducts have occurred. Pancreatitis due to an endoprosthesis has not been reported.

The frequency of dislodgement of the endoprostheses (3.5%) was not high in comparison with the 5% reported with external/internal drainage catheters (Burcharth 1982).

## Summary and Conclusion

Transhepatic insertion of an endoprosthesis for internal biliary drainage was attempted in 455 patients with obstructive jaundice. It was successful in 402 patients (88%), and 353 of these patients (88%) had permanent drainage with the endoprosthesis. Complications caused by the insertion occurred in 5.5% and late complications in 12.1%. Seven patients (1.5%) died as a result of complications. The plasma bilirubin level became normal in 188 of 283 patients (66%) with permanent endoprosthesis for malignant stenosis. The median survival time in patients with malignant lesions was 3.2 months with a range of less than one month to 3 years. Most of these patients had advanced cancer at the time of insertion.

The technique for transhepatic insertion of an endoprosthesis is relatively easy, and, as an alternative to surgery, seems to have little risk. The method may be used for temporary drainage before surgery; as emergency management of acute suppurative cholangitis, or for permanent drainage in patients with inoperable lesions; either benign or malignant, and in patients presenting a prohibitively high operative risk.

## Acknowledgments

Contributors to the data collected:

M. Adler and M. Cremer, Department of Gastroenterology, Hospital Erasme, Brussels, Belgium; F. Burcharth, Departments of Surgical Gastroenterology and Radiology, Herlev University Hospital, Copenhagen, Denmark; J. S. Dooley and R. Dick, Departments of Medicine and Radiology, Royal Free Hospital, London, England; J. T. Ferrucci Jr., Department of Radiology, Massachusetts General Hospital, Boston, USA; J. Hoevels, Institute of Clinical Radiology, Klinikum Mannheim, Mannheim, West Germany; S. Karlsson, Department of Radiology, General Hospital, Malmø, Sweden; G. A. D. McPherson and L. H. Blumgart, Hepatobiliary Unit, Hammersmith Hospital, London, England; J. F. Riemann and L. Demling, Department of Internal Medicine, University of Erlangen-Nuremberg, Erlangen, West Germany; and N. Rupp, Institute of Diagnostik Radiology, Technische Universität, Klinikum rechts der Isar, Munich, West Germany.

## References

Braasch JW, Gray BN (1977) Considerations that lower pancreatoduodenectomy mortality. Am J Surg 133:480–483

Burcharth F (1978) A new endoprosthesis for nonoperative intubation of the biliary tract in malignant obstructive jaundice. Surg Gynecol Obstet 146:76–78

Burcharth F (1982) Nonsurgical drainage of the biliary tract. Semin Liver Dis 2:75–86

Burcharth F, Nielbo N (1976) Percutaneous transhepatic cholangiography with selective catheterization of the common bile duct. AJR 127:409–412

Burcharth F, Pedersen JH (1981) Internal endoprosthesis as treatment of obstructive jaundice in pancreatitis. Fortschr Geb Röntgenstr Nuklearmed Ergänzungsband 134:290–293
Burcharth F, Christiansen L, Efsen F, Nielbo N, Stage P (1977) Percutaneous transhepatic cholangiography in diagnostic evaluation of 160 jaundiced patients. Results of an improved technique. Am J Surg 133:559–561
Burcharth F, Jensen LI, Olesen K (1979) Endoprosthesis for internal drainage of the biliary tract. Gastroenterology 77:133–137
Burcharth F, Efsen F, Christiansen LA, Hancke S, Jensen LI, Nielsen OV, Pedersen JH, Pedersen G (1981) Nonsurgical internal biliary drainage by endoprosthesis. Surg Gynecol Obstet 153:857–860
Denning DA, Ellison EC, Carey LC (1981) Preoperative percutaneous transhepatic biliary decompression lowers operative morbidity in patients with obstructive jaundice. Am J Surg 141:64
Dooley JS, Dick R, Olney J, Sherlock S (1979) Non-surgical treatment of biliary obstruction. Lancet II:1040–1043
Dooley JS, Dick R, Irving D, Olney J, Sherlock S (1981) Relief of bile duct obstruction by the percutaneous transhepatic insertion of an endoprosthesis. Clin Radiol 32:163–172
Feduska NJ, Dent TL, Lindenauer SM (1971) Results of palliative operations for carcinoma of the pancreas. Arch Surg 103:330–334
Ferrucci JT Jr, Mueller PR, Harbin WP (1980) Percutaneous transhepatic biliary drainage. Radiology 135:1–13
Glenn F, Evans JA, Muhajed Z, Thorbjarnarson B (1962) Percutaneous transhepatic cholangiography. Ann Surg 156:451–460
Hermann RE, Cooperman AM (1979) Current concepts in cancer. Cancer of the pancreas. N Engl J Med 301:482–485
Hoevels J, Ihse I (1979) Percutaneous transhepatic insertion of a permanent endoprosthesis in obstructive lesions of the extrahepatic bile ducts. Gastrointest Radiol 4:367–377
Hoevels J, Lunderquist A, Ihse I (1978) Perkutane transhepatische Intubation der Gallengänge zur kombinierten inneren und äußeren Drainage bei extrahepatischer Cholestase. Fortschr Geb Röntgenstr. Nuklearmed Ergänzungsband 129:533–550
Moden M, Okamura J, Kobayashi N, Shibata N, Horikawa S, Fujimoto T, Kosaki G, Kuroda C, Uchida H (1980) Hemobilia after percutaneous transhepatic biliary drainage. Arch Surg 115:161–164
Molnar W, Stockum E (1974) Relief of obstructive jaundice through percutaneous transhepatic catheter – A new therapeutic method. AJR 122:356–367
Mori K, Misumi A, Sugiyama M, Okabe M, Matsuoka T, Ishii J, Masanobu A (1977) Percutaneous transhepatic bile drainage. Ann Surg 185:111–115
Nakayama T, Ikeda A, Okuda K (1978) Percutaneous transhepatic drainage of the biliary tract. Gastroenterology 74:554–559
Okuda K, Musha H, Nakajima Y, Takayasu K, Suzuki Y, Morita M, Yamasaki T (1978) Frequency of intrahepatic arteriovenous fistula as a sequela to percutaneous needle puncture of the liver. Gastroenterology 74:1204–1207
Pereiras RV Jr, Reingold OJ, Hutson D, Mejia J, Viamonte M, Chiprut RO, Schiff ER (1978) Relief of malignant obstructive jaundice by percutaneous transhepatic insertion of a permanent prosthesis in the biliary tree. Ann Intern Med 89:589–593
Ring EJ, Oleaga J, Freiman DB, Husted JW, Lunderquist A (1978) Therapeutic applications of catheter cholangiography. Radiology 128:333–338
Rupp N, Weiss H-D (1980) Perkutan eingebrachte Gallengangsprothesen als Primärmaßnahme bei Verschlußikterus. Fortschr Geb Röntgenstr Nuklearmed Ergänzungsband 133:279–284
Takada T, Hanyu F, Kobayashi S, Uchida Y (1976) Percutaneous transhepatic cholangial drainage. Direct approach under fluoroscopic control. J Surg Oncol 8:83–97

# 9 Local Radiotherapy of Biliary Malignancies

*M. S. Fletcher, D. Brinkley, J. L. Dawson, H. Nunnerley, and Roger Williams*

## Introduction

Patients presenting with obstructive jaundice due to a cholangiocarcinoma involving the hilum of the liver pose a major problem in management. Despite recent advances in preoperative assessment of resectability and in operative techniques (Blumgart 1978; Williamson et al. 1980), in most reports the rate of attempted radical curative resection has remained very low (Inouye and Whelan 1978; Akwari and Kelly 1979; Evander et al. 1980; Blumgart 1982) and the operative mortality is still 10%–20% (Lannois et al. 1979; Evander et al. 1980). In contrast, effective palliation can often be achieved with low operative mortality if the obstruction is relieved by a cholangioenteric anastamosis (Cahow 1979) or by operative insertion of a transhepatic U tube (Terblanche et al. 1972).

With widespread acceptance of percutaneous transhepatic drainage as an established technique, satisfactory bile drainage can now be established in many patients before or as an alternative to surgery (Pollock et al. 1979; Nakayama et al. 1978; Hoevels et al. 1978; Dooley et al. 1981).

We have recently described a new method of providing localized internal radiotherapy using iridium 192-wire within the tumor itself once bile drainage has been established by means of either a transhepatic U tube or a percutaneous transhepatic catheter (Fletcher et al. 1981), and this paper reports our experience with this technique.

## Patients and Methods

Between June 1978 and March 1982, in all 18 patients with cholangiocarcinoma involving the hepatic hilus and 1 patient with carcinoma of the gallbladder causing common hepatic duct obstruction were treated with iridium-192 wire. There were 12 men and 7 women, with a mean age of 54.6 years (range 28–67).

Nine patients (47%) had had an initial laparotomy at another hospital before referral. Various different procedures were used in the initial management of these patients (Table 1). In the latter part of the series percutaneous transhepatic drainage was used if the cholangiographic appearances, supplemented in some cases by visceral angiography, indicated that the lesions were not resectable. In some patients satisfactory bile drainage was not obtained and further procedures were necessary (Table 2). Three patients had a further laparotomy and T tubes were replaced by transhepatic U tubes. In the remaining patients subsequent satisfactory placement of a percutaneous transhepatic catheter was performed.

The biliary system was allowed to decompress for 10–14 days before placement of the iridium-192 wire, as previously described (Fletcher et al. 1981). Radiation, calculated at a

**Table 1.** Primary procedure in 19 patients with obstructive jaundice due to carcinoma at the hilum of the liver

| Procedure | No. |
|---|---|
| Laparotomy and T tube | 7 |
| Laparotomy and U tube[a] | 5 |
| Laparotomy alone | 2 |
| Laparotomy and choledochojejunostomy | 1 |
| Percutaneous transhepatic drainage | 4 |
| Total | 19 |

[a] Three patients had preoperative percutaneous transhepatic drainage for 1–7 days

**Table 2.** Further procedures performed to obtain satisfactory bile drainage and iridium-192 wire placement

| Primary procedure | Subsequent procedure | No. |
|---|---|---|
| Laparotomy and T tube | Further laparotomy and U tube | 3 |
| Laparotomy and T tube | Percutaneous transhepatic catheter | 4 |
| Laparotomy alone | Percutaneous transhepatic catheter | 2 |
| Laparotomy alone and choledochojejunostomy | Percutaneous transhepatic catheter | 1 |
| Total | | 10 |

point 0.5 cm from the wire, was then given over a period of 40–48 h, after which the iridium wire was removed leaving the drainage catheter in place.

## Results

Nine of the 19 patients (47%) are still alive. Sixteen patients (84%) survived at least 6 months and 10 (52.6%) lived for 12 months or more, with an overall median survival of 11 months (range 4–38). Ten patients have died from the effects of tumor progression and biliary obstruction. Four patients have shown evidence (clinical or at postmortem) of distant spread of the disease.

Maintenance of bile drainage over prolonged periods has been a problem and tubes have required changing when they have become dislodged or blocked by biliary sludge or tumor recurrence.

Cholangitis has been the most common complication, and 9 patients (47%) have had positive bile cultures, usually with a mixture of organisms. One patient developed a bile-stained pleural effusion and another had a subhepatic bile collection noted at laparotomy following preoperative percutaneous bile drainage. Two patients developed a mucocele of the gallbladder owing to tumor progression causing obstruction of the cystic duct.

## Discussion

The value of radiotherapy or chemotherapy in the treatment of cholangiocarcinoma of the hilum of the liver has not yet been proved in a controlled prospective study, but these treatments seem to be of some value in patients in whom bile drainage has been achieved (Terblanche et al. 1982; Lees et al. 1980; Wheeler et al. 1981). Because external-beam radiotherapy requires prolonged patient attendance and may be complicated by damage to surrounding tissues, causing problems such as hemorrhagic gastritis and duodenal obstruction (Benjamin et al. 1981), we have advocated the use of internal radiotherapy with iridium-192 wire (Fletcher et al. 1981). This provides high-dosage radiation to the area around the wire, with a rapid tail-off a short distance from it. This minimizes the radiation damage to surrounding organs whilst ensuring that the maximum effect is directed at the central part of the tumor and in this way may delay progression of the tumor causing obstruction of drainage catheters.

Assessment of results is notoriously difficult in this condition, as the tumors are often slow-growing, and occasional long-term survivors are reported in most series. However, a median survival of 11 months with 10 patients (52.6%) surviving for 12 months or longer is very encouraging. With a technique of cholangio-enteric anastamosis, Cahow reported a "mean" survival of 16 months, but with a 21% operative mortality, and Lamois et al. (1979), Evander et al. (1980), and Blumgart (1982), who all advocate radical resection, have reported mean survivals of 14, 20, and 24 months, respectively, but with an operative mortality of about 20%. Mornex et al. (1981), using a similar technique to ours but with higher doses, have reported similar results and suggested that because of the rapid fall-off in radiation dose around the wire a combination of external-beam radiotherapy followed by internal radiotherapy with iridium-192 wire should be used.

The complications reported in this series seem to be related to the placement and maintenance of drainage tubes rather than the use of iridium itself. The frequent occurrence of cholangitis is related to the presence of external drainage and might thus be reduced by conversion to internal drainage with insertion of an endoprosthesis following iridium wire treatment.

Thus, this method of treatment may offer some benefit in terms of prolonging survival in those patients in whom bile drainage has been established. A prospective study is needed to assess the benefit compared with that derived from drainage alone and the value of differing dosage regimens.

## Summary

Eighteen patients with a cholangiocarcinoma involving the hilum of the liver and one patient with a carcinoma of the gallbladder causing obstruction of the common hepatic duct have been treated with bile drainage using a U tube (8 patients) or a percutaneous transhepatic catheter (11 patients) followed by internal radiotherapy with iridium-192 wire. The median survival is 11 months, and ten patients (52.6%) have survived for 12 months or longer.

These results suggest that the addition of internal radiotherapy may be beneficial in patients with hilar cholangiocarcinoma causing obstruction in whom bile drainage can be established.

## Acknowledgments

We thank Mr B. J. Morley, Department of Medical Physics, King's College Hospital, for his technical assistance.

## References

Akwari OE, Kelly KA (1979) Surgical treatment of adenocarcinoma: location junction of right and left and common hepatic biliary ducts. Arch Surg 114:22–25

Benjamin IS, McPherson GAD, Blumgart LH (1981) Iridium 192 wire for hilar cholangiocarcinoma. Lancet II:582–583

Blumgart LH (1978) Biliary tract obstruction: new approaches to old problems. Am J Surg 135:19–31

Blumgart HL (1982) New perspectives and old problems in biliary surgery. Surg News 13:1–4

Cahow CE (1979) Intrahepatic cholangiojejunostomy: a new simplified approach. Am J Surg 137:443–448

Dooley J, Dick R, Irving D, Olney J, Sherlock S (1981) Relief of bile duct obstruction by the percutaneous transhepatic insertion of an endoprosthesis. Clin Radiol 32:163–172

Evander A, Fredlund P, Hoevels J, Ihse I, Bengmark S (1980) Evaluation of aggressive surgery for carcinoma of the extrahepatic bile ducts. Ann Surg 191:23–29

Fletcher MS, Brinkley D, Dawson JL, Nunnerley H, Wheeler PG, Williams R (1981) The treatment of high bile ducts carcinoma by internal radiotherapy with iridium 192 wire. Lancet II:172–174

Hoevels J, Lunderquist A, Ihse I (1978) Percutaneous transhepatic intubation of bile ducts for combined internal – external drainage in peroperative and palliative treatment of obstructive jaundice. Gastrointest Radiol 3:23–31

Inouye AA, Whelan TJ (1978) Carcinoma of the extrahepatic bile ducts. A ten year experience in Hawaii. Am J Surg 136:90–95

Lamois B, Campion J-P, Brissot P (1979) Carcinoma of the hepatic hilus. Ann Surg 190:151–157

Lees CD, Zapolanski A, Cooperman AM, Hermann PE (1980) Carcinoma of the bile ducts. Surg Gynaecol Obstet 151:193–198

Mornex F, Gerard J-P, Bret P, Partensky P (1981) Iridium wire radiotherapy for high bile duct carcinoma. Lancet II:479

Nakayama T, Ikeda A, Okukda K (1978) Percutaneous transhepatic drainage of the biliary tract. Gastroenterology 74:554–559

Pollock TW, Ring ER, Oleaga JA, Freiman DB, Mullen JL, Rosato EF (1979) Percutaneous decompression of benign and malignant biliary obstruction. Arch Surg 114:148–151

Terblanche J, Saunders SJ, Louw JH (1972) Prolonged palliation in carcinoma of the main hepatic duct junction. Surgery 71:720–731

Wheeler PG, Dawson JL, Nunnerley H, Brinkley D, Laws J, Williams R (1981) Newer techniques in the diagnosis and treatment of proximal bile duct carcinoma – an analysis of 41 consecutive cases. Q J Med 50:247–259

Williamson BWA, Blumgart LH, McKellar NJ (1980) The management of tumours of the liver. Am J Surg 139:210–215

# 10 Preoperative Biliary Drainage: A Controlled Trial

*A. R. W. Hatfield and J. Terblanche*

## Perioperative Management

The total management of the jaundiced patient has improved significantly recently, resulting in diminished morbidity and increased survival of patients undergoing operative procedures for obstructive jaundice. It is important to recognize this in evaluating new forms of treatment, which must be tested in prospective randomized trials. They should not be compared with historical controls who underwent operation at an earlier date when both morbidity and mortality were higher.

The current perioperative management of jaundiced patients in Cape Town includes measures to improve the general condition of the patient. However, the important aspects of the improved recent management include the use of perioperative antibiotics, and a better understanding of hydration. Studies from our laboratory by Bailey (Bailey 1976) indicated that jaundiced patients developed endotoxaemia and decreased creatinine clearance when their bilirubin was greater than 144.5 μmol/liter (8.5 mg per 100 ml). In a separate rat study Bailey noted that bile duct ligation produced endotoxemia and that this was eliminated by administering bile salts (Bailey 1976). He concluded that endotoxin played a role in the pathogenesis of renal failure in jaundiced patients. Similar conclusions with regard to the possible role of endotoxin in the pathogenesis of renal failure in jaundiced patients were reached by the group at King's College Hospital, London, in a study of 45 patients with cirrhosis and 12 patients with obstructive jaundice (Wilkinson et al. 1976). Our group believes that perioperative antibiotics reduce the endotoxemia and increase the creatinine clearance in jaundiced patients. In addition, short-term antibiotic cover should be utilized in patients who have obstructive jaundice and who undergo invasive investigations of the biliary tree.

The important factor in maintaining hydration is adequate perioperative intravenous fluid administration. Dawson (1965) drew attention to the importance of adequate urine flow in the management of jaundiced patients. He used mannitol 10% (Dawson 1965). Subsequently others have used frusemide to ensure urine flow, but it is the authors' contention that the most important aspect of management is to provide an adequate fluid load. Most patients will then secrete sufficient urine and maintain good renal function. Frusemide and/or mannitol are only administered to patients who fail to pass adequate amounts of urine in the perioperative period despite a fluid load. The authors' group favors frusemide in this setting. An adequate fluid load is also important in patients undergoing invasive investigations of the biliary tree.

In addition, preoperative PTC and/or ERCP have assisted in the perioperative management of jaundiced patients. One or both can provide a diagnosis and a route map for the surgeon. Both the surgeon and the anesthetist are then prepared for either major or minor surgery, depending on the lesion and the current policy of management of that particular lesion.

## Preoperative Biliary Drainage

Preoperative biliary drainage can be established via either PTC or ERC, and has been shown to significantly diminish the serum bilirubin of jaundiced patients (Nakayama et al. 1978). This has been extrapolated to the modern management of patients with obstructive jaundice, and it has been concluded that improved survival and diminished morbidity would result if preoperative biliary drainage were instituted. Unfortunately, all the data on which this conclusion is based eminate from uncontrolled trials of sequential groups of patients. This criticism has been discussed earlier. Probably the most widely quoted paper ist that of Nakayama et al. (1978). Others have reached a similar conclusion, also based on uncontrolled trials (Tylen et al. 1977; Hansson et al. 1979). In 1979 Dooley suggested that a prospective randomized controlled trial would be needed to prove this point (Dooley et al. 1979), but to date no such trials have been published.

The technical problems and complications of preoperative biliary drainage are more common than is generally perceived. The first question is how long biliary drainage should be continued. In many series a period of 1–2 weeks has been utilized, by which time the bilirubin, if very high, has usually dropped by at least 50%. However, Koyama et al. (1981) have pointed out that a period of at least 4–6 weeks' biliary drainage is probably necessary to obtain improvement in mitochondrial respiratory function, ketogenesis, and the return to normal of altered collagen metabolism. If the patient has been jaundiced for over 6 weeks the period of biliary drainage may need to be as long as 12 weeks. On the other hand, Blenkharn and co-workers (Blenkharn et al. 1981) have pointed out that, unless one has a completely closed system of biliary drainage, infection is introduced into the biliary tree within 4 days of the introduction of the percutaneous transhepatic catheter. This in itself creates new problems for the patients, and might even result in diminished renal function, particularly if hydration is not adequately maintained during this period. In addition, there are specific complications, including biliary leakage into both the peritoneal cavity and the pleural cavity and hemorrhage, which are not insignificant in the types of patients being discussed. A final potential problem is one that occurs for the surgeon who is used to handling the thin-walled dilated proximal bile ducts and is now faced with collapsed bile ducts which are small. However, drained ducts tend to have a thicker wall and are not difficult to handle surgically.

### *Cape Town Trial*

Preliminary data are available from a prospective randomized controlled trial of preoperative biliary drainage undertaken in Cape Town (Hatfield et al. 1982). A total of 57 patients were entered into the trial, all of whom had a serum bilirubin greater than 150 μmol/liter.

Twenty-nine were randomized to the drainage group and 28 to the no-drainage group. After initial exclusions 25 and 27 patients remained in the two groups, respectively. In the drainage group the serum bilirubin fell from a mean of 360 μmol/liter to 134 μmol/liter in the 12-day (average) period of drainage. In the no-drainage group the mean serum bilirubin level was 320 μmol/liter.

Of the 25 patients who were randomized to drainage, 22 were submitted to laparotomy, while 25 of the 27 no-drainage patients were submitted to laparotomy. All had perioperative systemic antibiotics and a fluid load. They proved to have similar pathology and the postoperative complications related to the surgery itself were equal in the two groups. Three patients in the drainage group developed renal failure, 2 of these preoperatively during the phase of biliary drainage. No patient in the no-drainage group developed renal failure, in the perioperative period. The major problem in this group of patients was the significant incidence of drainage complications in those undergoing biliary drainage, even though the senior author, Hatfield, had had experience of this technique in the past (Hatfield and Murray 1981). In this group, in addition, bile became infected in 11, but in only 1 was this significant for the overall management of the patient. Perioperative mortality was 12% (3 of 25) in the drainage group and 15% (4 of 27) in the no-drainage group. There were 1 immediate postoperative surgical death in the drainage group and 2 in the no-drainage group (Hatfield et al. 1982).

It has been concluded that preoperative biliary drainage significantly diminishes the serum bilirubin, but that the perioperative morbidity and mortality are not reduced. In addition, preoperative biliary drainage has introduced significant morbidity in otherwise fit jaundiced patients. The justification for the routine use of preoperative biliary drainage must therefore be questioned as a result of this prospective randomized controlled clinical trial (Hatfield et al. 1982). The results of other prospective trials are awaited with interest.

## References

Bailey ME (1976) Endotoxin, bile salts and renal function in obstructive jaundice. Br J Surg 63:774–778

Blenkharn JI, McPherson GAD, Blumgart LH (1981) An improved system for external biliary drainage. Lancet 2:781–782

Dawson JL (1965) Postoperative renal function in obstructive jaundice: Effect of a Mannitol diuresis. Br Med J 1:82–86

Dooley JS, Dick R, Olney J, Sherlock S (1979) Non-surgical treatment of biliary obstruction. Lancet 2:1040–1044

Hansson JA, Hoevels J, Simert G, Tylen U, Vang J (1979) Clinical aspects of nonsurgical percutaneous transhepatic bile drainage in obstructive lesions of the extrahepatic bile ducts. Ann Surg 189:58–61

Hatfield ARW, Murray RS (1981) Pre-operative biliary drainage in patients with obstructive jaundice. A comparison of the percutaneous transhepatic and endoscopic transpapillary routes. S Afr Med J 60:737–742

Hatfield AR, Tobias R, Terblanche J, Girdwood AH, Fataar S, Harries-Jones R, Schulman A, Kernoff L, Marks IN (1982) Pre-operative external biliary drainage in obstructive jaundice. A prospective controlled clinical trial. Lancet 2:896–899

Koyama K, Takagi Y, Ito K, Sato T (1981) Experimental and clinical studies on the effect of biliary drainage in obstructive jaundice. Am J Surg 142:293–299

Nakayama T, Ikeda A, Okuda K (1978) Percutaneous transhepatic drainage of the biliary tract. Technique and results in 104 cases. Gastroenterology 74:554–559

Tylen U, Hoevels J, Vang J (1977) Percutaneous transhepatic cholangiography with external drainage of obstructive biliary lesions. Surg Gynec Obstet 144:13–18

Wilkinson SP, Moodie H, Stamatakis JD, Kakkar VV, Williams R (1976) Endotoxaemia and renal failure in cirrhosis and obstructive jaundice. Brit Med J 2:1415–1418

# 11 Percutaneous Bile Drainage: Discussion, Summary

*J. Dooley*

Percutaneous transhepatic biliary drainage has developed during the last 10 years from a specialist procedure carried out in a few centers to a form of therapy performed in many district general hospitals. Few comparisons of the techniques used and the results obtained have been published, however. The symposium provided an opportunity to review the percutaneous procedures and to compare the techniques and results. This summary attempts to outline the areas of agreement and disagreement among the participants of the round table.

Bile duct catheterization is the initial step for all the transhepatic procedures. It may be followed by intraperitoneal bile leakage and hemorrhage, hemobilia, and sepsis, and the overall incidence of major complications reported by Riemann was approximately 7%. Although many modifications in technique have been advocated as being safer, a major factor which influences the incidence of complications is the experience of the operator. In Riemann's review, centers which had treated fewer patients had a higher complication rate. Differences in technique also have some influence, and Nakayama et al. reported a lower risk when real-time ultrasound was used rather than fluoroscopy to visualize the bile ducts during the insertion of the catheter through the liver and into duct (12% vs 3%). Discussion of these data, however, indicated that most centers will continue to use x-ray screening, because of the relative lack of ultrasound equipment and expertise available in the x-ray suite. Also fluoroscopy would still be needed to screen subsequent guide wire and catheter manipulations within the bile ducts. Lateral x-ray screening was not thought to be necessary for bile duct catheterization by the majority of the discussion panel.

The position and number of ducts catheterized is a major area of controversy. Scandinavian working groups advocate catheterization of two bile ducts. The peripheral, usually dorsocaudal, duct is used for manipulation of the endoprosthesis or other equipment, while the other duct is used for decompression of the system and injection of contrast agent. Burcharth and our own unit normally catheterize only one duct, often central rather than peripheral. Interestingly, Riemann reported, from his review, that there appeared to be fewer complications in the centers using the two-catheter approach.

The argument against the use of a central or perihilar duct for manipulations of large catheters and endoprostheses is the proximity of major blood vessels which may be damaged. Puncture of a peripheral duct, however, may result in a more tortuous path through the biliary system to the common bile duct, and a shorter thickness of liver to seal the track between bile duct and peritoneal cavity. Further comparisons of these two approaches would be valuable.

There was no clear consensus of opinion, and no information, to support the use of antibiotic premedication in patients *without* a clinical suspicion of biliary infection.

External bile drainage has been advocated for the preoperative preparation of deeply jaundiced patients. This approach has been criticised because of the lack of evidence of benefit, and also because of the problems due to the loss of bile. The first randomized controlled trial of benefit, reported by Hatfield and Terblanche at this meeting, compared postoperative mortality and morbidity in patients with and without preoperative external bile drainage. No difference was detected between the groups. This trial was criticised because of the small number of patients studied, and therefore lack of statistical confidence in the certainty of the conclusions. From the practical viewpoint, even if a further trial were to show benefit from preoperative external bile drainage, this would have to be weighed against the risks of such treatment. Although Hofmann did not foresee any dangers from the short-term loss of the organic constituents of bile, the loss of water and sodium can cause dehydration. Also colonization of the biliary system with bacteria may produce septic complications. The panel agreed that preoperative external bile drainage by the percutaneous route is not indicated on the present evidence.

Whether selected patients with acute suppurative cholangitis should be treated initially by nonsurgical decompression by the percutaneous or transpapillary route in combination with antibiotics has not been studied under trial conditions, but Terblanche thought that this was potentially the best management. Trials are still needed to test the effect of preoperative drainage in patients with potentially resectable malignant lesions. Thus, the only group of patients in whom external drainage remains of undisputed value is that in whom surgery and other interventional techniques cannot provide internal bile drainage. However, even in this group any symptomatic benefit (i.e., loss of itching) must be judged against possible lowering of the quality of life due to the external tube.

Catheterization of strictures, malignant or benign, to provide internal drainage of bile is now possible by the percutaneous transhepatic route in 90%–95% of patients. Internal/external drainage has not been as popular in Europe as in the United States, possibly because of the success of endoprostheses in Europe. However, internal/external tubes have the distinct advantage of allowing easy access to the drainage catheter for flushing or exchange. Pereiras pointed out that the tubes used should be of wide bore (Fr. 12 or 14) with wide side-holes. The present use of Fr. 7–8 catheters with smaller side holes has probably been responsible for the problems of sepsis, and in his patients the incidence of "delayed" complications was reduced from 30% to 2% by increasing the tube diameter to Fr. 12.

The alternative approach for internal bile drainage is the endoprosthesis. The overall incidence of complications of insertion in Burcharth's review was 5%, and the factors governing these have as far as possible been discussed under "catheterization" above. The optimal shape and diameter of the tube, size and number of side holes, and type of plastic used, are controversial. Both large- and small-bore tubes relieve jaundice in a similar percentage of patients, and both may become filled with debris. However, obstruction to bile flow due to blockage of the tube has not been a problem in patients with malignant disease, who generally have a poor prognosis and a short survival. Although there was disagreement regarding the optimal diameter of the endoprosthesis, most agreed that the shape and length of the tube should be chosen according to the anatomy of each biliary system. Thus in some patients the use of preformed commercial tubes may lead to inadequate drainage of bile.

A major topic which escaped discussion at the symposium was the selection of patients for endoprosthesis rather than for surgery. Although some patients have obviously irresectable disease with metastases, in others the picture is less clearcut. Although Arnesjö suggested that laparotomy alone could rule out resectability, more practical guidelines based on the combination of data from scanning, cholangiography, laparoscopy, and angiography are needed.

Radiotherapy for cholangiocarcinoma, using a radioactive wire placed through the stricture within a transhepatic tube, is an attractive addition to the sparse therapeutic choice for cholangiocarcinoma. The results reported by Fletcher are difficult to evaluate in the absence of controlled data, but a randomized trial with a large number of patients with known histology would be virtually impossible to perform. However, perhaps a multicenter trial should be encouraged before widespread use of this technique.

The more erudite transhepatic techniques, such as stone removal and cholangioscopy, have a place in the management of a minority of patients, but should probably be restricted to the centers that have particular expertise available.

In conclusion, percutaneous transhepatic drainage techniques have become part of the therapeutic choice for patients with obstructive jaundice. External bile drainage, although easier to perform than internal drainage, lacks data supporting its use before surgery. The major role of these techniques for the future appears to be to provide internal bile drainage. Evidence of statistical benefit of this approach compared with surgery does not yet exist, but in the absence of an unacceptably high incidence of complications, it has a role in place of palliative surgery in selected patients. In the future, refinements of technique and equipment should reduce complications and increase success, and we must welcome opportunities to discuss individual variations in approach to achieve this end.

# III. The Transpapillary Approach

# 12 Techniques of Endoscopic Bile Drainage

*K. Huibregtse*

Since the first description of a method to insert a biliary endoprosthesis through a fiberendoscope (Soehendra and Reynders-Frederix 1979) a rapid development of various endoprostheses and techniques of introducing them has taken place.

## Endoprosthesis

Initially an angiographic catheter with one pigtail end and 12 side-holes was used. The pigtail served to avoid dislodgement towards the duodenum. Because in some patients with a distal stenosis and extremely dilated bile ducts dislodgement above the stenosis into the dilated bile ducts was observed, the double-pigtail catheter was developed (Fig. 1). Dislodgement of this endoprosthesis is rare. The double-pigtail catheter is available in 5, 7, and 9 French, 15 cm long, and is made of teflon tubing.

A disadvantage of the pigtail catheter is that especially in bifurcation tumors when the intrahepatic bile ducts are not dilated, the pigtail does not develop. Therefore we developed a straight endoprosthesis with many side-holes and two side-flaps to avoid dislodgement. In 250 patients, only in one patient with a malignant stenosis has dislodgement of such an endoprosthesis been seen. Depend-

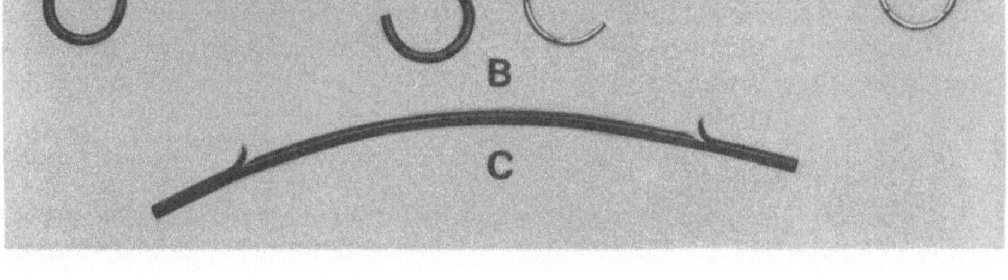


**Fig. 1.** *A* pigtail endoprosthesis; *B* double pig-tail endoprosthesis; *C* straight endoprosthesis with sideflaps

ing on the site of the stenosis a 15- or 20-cm-long endoprosthesis is used. The straight endoprosthesis is made of Fr. 7 or 9 polyethylene tubing (Fig. 1).

Further advantages of the straight endoprosthesis over the pigtail type are easier introduction, because less friction is encountered when the prosthesis is slid over the guide wire, and the absence of trauma to the common duct or duodenal wall. In 250 patients no such traumata were observed. Common duct perforations have occurred with pigtail catheters.

### *Development of Technique*

In the first description a papillotomy was first performed to facilitate introduction of the endoprosthesis. A side-viewing endoscope was then loaded with the pigtail endoprosthesis straightened over a metal guide wire. The endoscope was introduced and the straightened endoprosthesis was pushed through and beyond the stenosis by a pusher catheter. Introduction of the straightened endoprosthesis must be successful at the first attempt. Once the endoprosthesis is pushed out of the endoscope it is impossible to withdraw it into the endoscope and to try a second time. The endoscope must be removed and the endoprosthesis pushed into the instrumentation channel for a second trial. To avoid this problem it is easier to maneuver a catheter with a guide wire inside through and beyond the stenosis. The catheter is removed, leaving the guide wire in place. The endoprosthesis is pushed into position over the guide wire by a pusher catheter.

The maximum outside diameter of the endoprosthesis is limited and depends on the inside diameter of the instrumentation channel of the available endoscope. The initial experience with the Fr. 5 and 7 endoprostheses included a large number of cholangitis complications. This complication was believed to be due partly to inaccurate disinfection of the endoscope, and partly to the relatively small caliber of the endoprosthesis, not allowing free bile drainage. Several techniques and instruments have been developed to insert larger-caliber endoprostheses (Huibregtse et al. 1981a, b; 1982a, b). These techniques will not be described here, because they have become history with the introduction of the prototype duodenoscope with a 3.7-mm instrumentation channel (Fig. 2). With this endoscope a Fr. 9 endoprosthesis can easily be introduced.

Proper disinfection of the endoscope and the ancillary equipment is mandatory. Cholangitis after insertion of a 9 Fr. endoprosthesis allowing good drainage ought to be a rare exception. In patients with a bifurcation tumor, in whom only one liver lobe can be drained, however, cholangitis occurs frequently in the non-drained lobe even after proper disinfection of the equipment. Sometimes in these cases cholangitis can only be successfully treated by introduction of an endoprosthesis in the other lobe as well.

### *Established Technique*

First an ERCP is performed to obtain information on the biliary and pancreatic anatomy. An endoscopic papillotomy is performed to facilitate the introduction of the various catheters. It is also believed that a papillotomy lowers the risk of pancreatitis by avoiding occlusion of the pancreatic duct by the endoprosthesis.

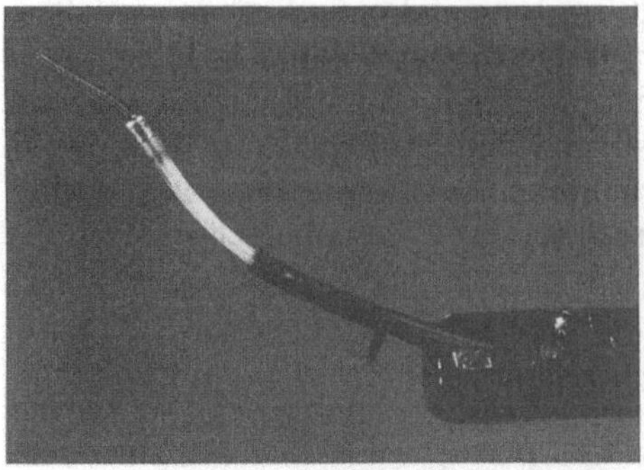

**Fig. 2.** Tip of prototype Olympus duodenoscope with 3.7-mm instrumentation channel. The endoscope is loaded with a straight Fr. 9 endoprosthesis over a 2.1-mm catheter with metal tip, with an atraumatic guide wire inside

Using the 2.8-mm instrumentation channel endoscope, a 2.1-mm teflon catheter with a 4-m-long atraumatic guide wire inside is pushed through and beyond the stenosis. In case of failure the stenosis is first passed by the guide wire and then the catheter is pushed over the guide wire through the stenosis. Firm stenoses, which are difficult to pass, must be dilated with stiff teflon catheters of increasing diameter up to the diameter of the endoprosthesis before positioning of the endoprosthesis. Once the catheter with the guide wire inside has passed the stenosis the catheter is removed, leaving the guide wire in place. The endoprosthesis is pushed over the guide wire to beyond the stenosis by a pusher catheter of the same diameter. During the introduction of the endoprosthesis through the instrumentation channel the tip of the endoscope must be kept close to the papilla, and care must be taken that the guide wire is not pushed forward into the duodenal lumen allowing it to slip out the common duct into the duodenum. Using the prototype jumbo-duodenoscope with a 3.7-mm channel the straight Fr. 9 endoprosthesis must be inserted over the rather stiff 2.1-mm catheter with the guide wire inside, largely avoiding the above-mentioned risk of the guide wire slipping out of the common duct. All pigtail endoprostheses must be inserted over the metal guide wire. After positioning of the endoprosthesis the guide wire is withdrawn, while the endoprosthesis is kept in place by the pusher tube. In case of a pigtail endoprosthesis the curl in the tail develops. The endoprosthesis is pushed out of the endoscope. The distal end of the endoprosthesis hangs free in the duodenum and the endoscope is removed. It is preferable to have the distal end of the endoprosthesis protruding in the duodenal lumen. For removal of the endoprosthesis in case of clogging, the distal end can easily be grasped by a foreign body remover, polypectomy snare, or dormia basket. Before introduction of the straight endoprosthesis with two barbed hooks into the instrumentation channel, the cap of the instrumentation channel must be unscrewed and removed. A short piece of tubing with the same internal diameter as the instrumentation channel must be used to press the lower barbed hook into the instrumentation channel.

## Discussion

The technique for introduction of biliary stents is now well established and for endoscopists familiar with ERCP and endoscopic papillotomy it is an easy procedure. In general the entire procedure takes no more than 30–45 minutes. The

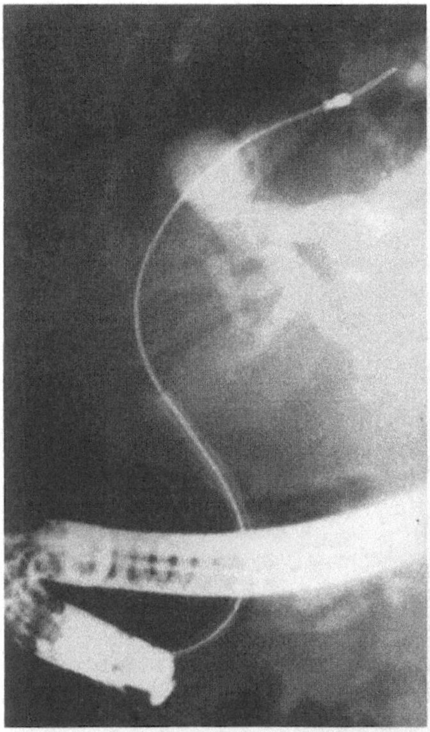

a

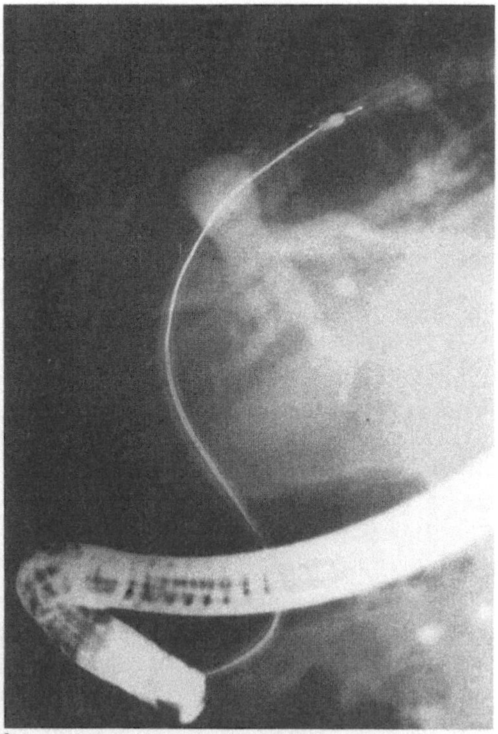

b

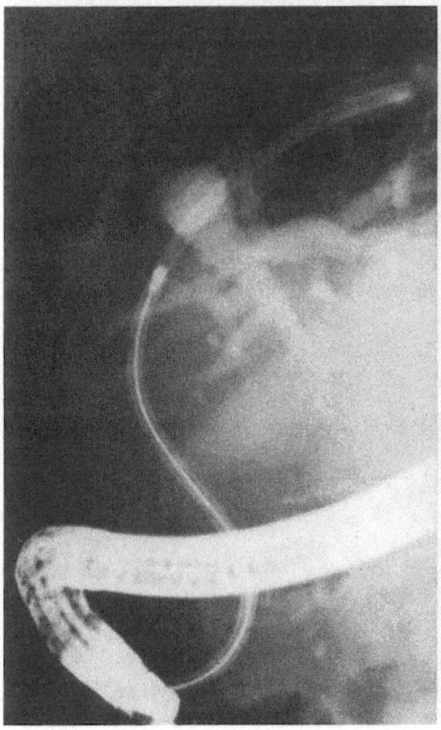

c

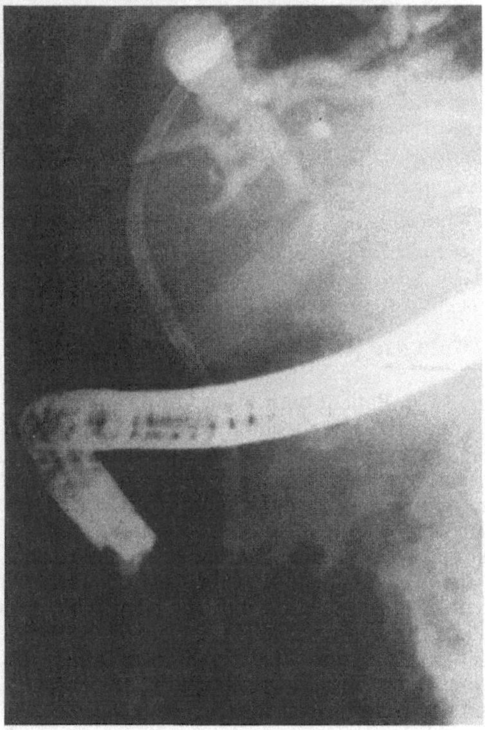

d

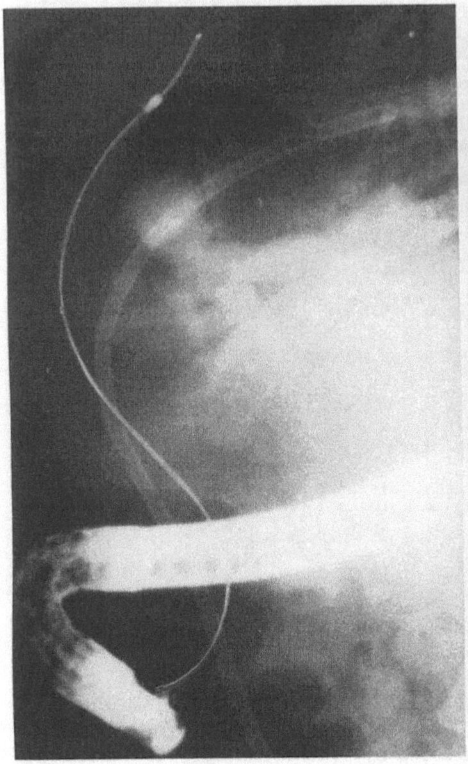

e

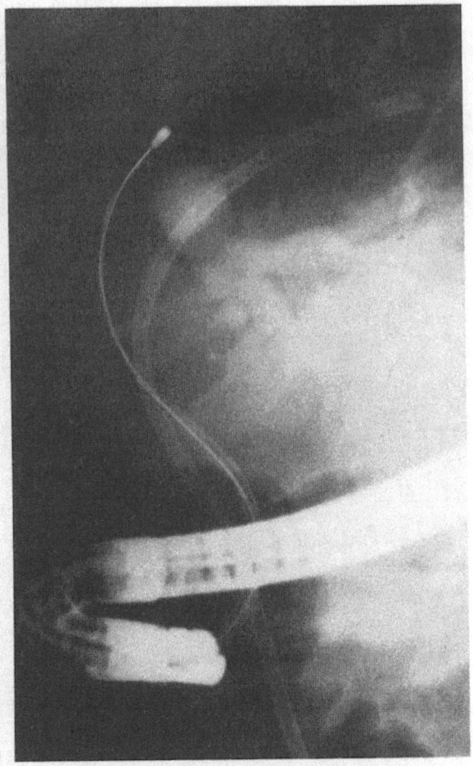

f

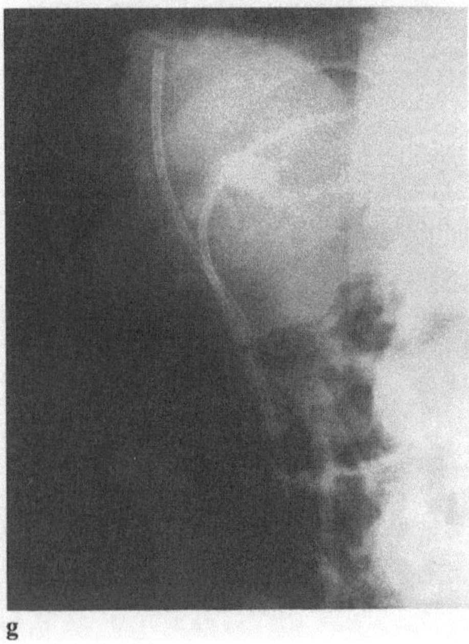

g

**Fig. 3 a–g.** Patient with bifurcation tumor. **a** The catheter and guide wire above the stenosis; **b** the endoprosthesis is pushed into the left liver lobe; **c** catheter and guide wire are removed, leaving the endoprosthesis in place, by pushing the pusher catheter; **d** the endoprosthesis free in the duodenum; **e** catheter and guide wire beyond the stenosis and extending into the right liver lobe; **f** the endoprosthesis is advanced over the catheter into the right liver lobe; **g** one endoprosthesis positioned in the left and one in right liver lobe

papillotomy is frequently the most time-consuming step of the procedure. Separate cannulation and papillotomy is difficult, because there is no bile flow and a normal papilla seems to be more difficult to cannulate than a papilla in the case of common duct stones. A precut of the papilla before proper papillotomy is necessary in a great percentage of the patients (Wurbs 1982).

The second most time-consuming step of the procedure is the maneuvering of the guide wire and catheter through the stenosis. In pancreatic cancer and middle common duct obstructions this is mostly no problem. In periampullary cancers and in bifurcation tumors it can be extremely difficult, and many attempts may be needed before it is successfully accomplished.

Further research must be directed at the development of devices to facilitate insertion of an endoprosthesis to drain both liver lobes in case of liver hilum tumors. Furthermore, the field of endoscopic stents must be extended to the pancreatic duct in cases of distal obstructions due to chronic pancreatitis or pancreatic cancer.

## References

Huibregtse K, Tytgat GN (1982a) Palliative treatment of obstructive jaundice by transpapillary introduction of a large bore bile duct endoprosthesis. Gut 23:371–375

Huibregtse K, Tytgat GN (1982b) Endoscopic drainage of biliary tract obstructions. In: Kawai K (ed) Frontiers of Gl endoscopy. Olympus Optical, pp 39–42

Huibregtse K, Haverkamp HJ, Tytgat GN (1981a) Transpapillary positioning of a large 3.2 mm biliary endoprosthesis. Endoscopy 13:217–219

Huibregtse K, Haverkamp HJ, Tytgat GN (1981b) Transpapillary introduced large bore bile duct endoprosthesis in the palliative treatment of malignant jaundice. Proceedings of Stomach Diseases. Excerpta Medica, Amsterdam, pp 135–142

Soehendra N, Reynders-Frederix V (1979) Palliative Gallengangdrainage. Dtsch Med Wschr 104:206–207

Soehendra N, Reynders-Frederix V (1980) Palliative bile duct drainage – a new endoscopic method of introducing a transpapillary drain. Endoscopy 12:8–11

Wurbs D (1982) Endoscopic papillotomy: In: Quadrennial reviews of the world congresses of gastroenterology and digestive endoscopy. Sweden, pp 107–115

# 13 Results of Bilionasal Drainage

*D. Wurbs*

The technique of continuous choledochal catheterization with a bilionasal tube was first used by Nagai et al. in 1976 . This technique using a Teflon tube has recently been applied in repeated cholangiography after endoscopic sphincterotomy for common bile duct stones (Cotton et al. 1979). These Teflon tubes become dislocated at a rate of 26% (Cotton et al. 1979) to 50% (Nagai et al. 1976). This high frequency of dislocation is not acceptable in the treatment of high-risk conditions which require reliable drainage of the bile ducts. Balloon catheters (Shapiro and Cotton 1975) may be fixed securely in the bile duct, but they have the disadvantage of a small inner diameter; they may obstruct the bile duct and are very expensive. We have developed a simple and effective method of bilionasal drainage using a self-fixing catheter of thermoplastic material of our own design which is inserted through the endoscope (Wurbs and Classen 1977). The distal end of the catheter has a special configuration which adapts to the normal anatomy of the duodenum and bile duct (Figs. 1 and 2). The outer diameter is 2.2 mm, and the length 1.8 m; the catheter volume is 2.8 ml. An endoscope with a 2.5 to 2.8-mm-diameter channel is needed for insertion of the tube.

The first step in introducing the tube is to move an impacted stone into the proximal aspect of the bile duct. This may be difficult, but with the rigid catheter some force can be exerted. The second step is to pass the tip of the catheter beyond the stone. This may also be difficult, however a soft and thin mandrin Seldinger

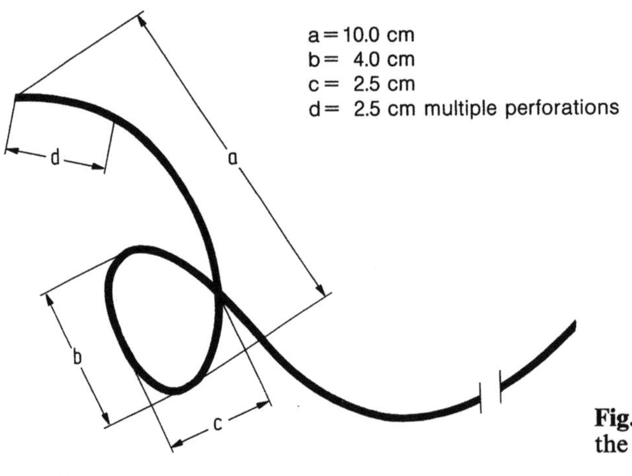


**Fig. 1.** Size and configuration of the self-fixing bilionasal tube

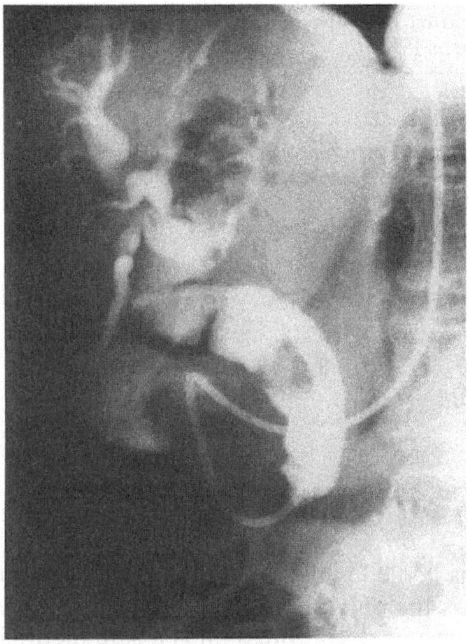

**Fig. 2.** The self-fixing bilionasal tube in situ. The tip has passed the stone and the tube thus preventing the impaction or reimpaction of the stone

type wire can serve as a guide. This guide wire is also helpful in passing a malignant stricture. When the tip of the catheter has reached the correct position at the hepatic junction, the endoscope is slowly withdrawn under fluoroscopic control. Simultaneously, the bilionasal tube is advanced in the instrument channel to match each length of instrument withdrawn until the instrument emerges from the mouth leaving the catheter in place. Finally, the tube is rerouted through the nose. The indwelling tube prevents reimpaction of the stone and thus guarantees a free flow of the bile to the duodenum. Bile may be aspirated through the drain at any time, and x-ray contrast medium or drugs, such as agents for dissolving stones, may be flushed into the bile duct. In our experience with more than 100 cases, the tube is well tolerated for many days or even weeks.

Suppurative cholangitis in association with bile duct obstruction has been a major complication (Classen et al. 1979) of endoscopic papillotomy. The need for endoscopic decompression of the bile ducts has been the motivating factor for the development of this bilionasal tube (Wurbs and Classen 1977). However, it has also been found to be useful in the following circumstances:

1. Decompression of obstructed bile duct
2. Prevention of stone impaction after endoscopic papillotomy
3. Treatment of a bilicutaneous fistula
4. Dissolution of common duct stones
5. Aspiration of bile for chemical and bacteriological study
6. Bile drainage through malignant stricture of the bile duct.

**Table 1.** Results of decompression of the bile duct in acute obstructive suppurative cholangitis. (After Wurbs 1982)

| Decompression | Died | |
|---|---|---|
| | Whole group | Operated group |
| Surgical | 34/82 (41%) | 19/67 (28%) |
| Endoscopic | 4/19 (21%) | 4/19 (21%) |

[a] Differences not significant in $\chi^2$-test

## Decompression of Obstructed Bile Ducts

Acute obstructive suppurative cholangitis is the highly dangerous extreme form of bacterial cholangitis. Until recent years the only alternative in treatment has been surgical decompression. Now, endoscopic decompression is a safe method of decompression of the common bile duct which has reduced risk compared with surgery even in extremely sick and old (mean age 81 years) patients (Wurbs 1982) (Table 1). About a quarter of the patients in collected surgical series were regarded as inoperable. These patients died without exception. Endoscopic decompression is not restricted by age, other severe disease, or even sepsis with associated coagulopathy and mental confusion.

The introduction and correct positioning of the bilionasal tube was achieved in all cases without complication after a very small endoscopic papillotomy (EPT). Drainage was adequate in all cases except one. Temperature normalized within a few hours, and pathological laboratory data (leucocytosis, GPT, alkaline phosphatase, bilirubin) returned to normal within a few days. Further therapy, endoscopic or surgical, may be carried out 7–10 days later as the second part of a two-step procedure.

The results of endoscopic retrograde drainage can be considered good when compared with surgical treatment (Table 1). The mortality in endoscopic retrograde drainage is approximately the same as that in early operated cases (21% vs. 28%), but is less in endoscopic drainage when all patients in both groups are compared (21% vs. 41%), and also less if elderly patients are considered (the difference being more than 10 years between surgically and endoscopically treated patients).

## Prevention of Stone Impaction

Large stones which are not extractable tend to impact after endoscopic papillotomy. An in situ bilionasal tube will reliably prevent this complication. Therefore, further therapy may be planned in an elective manner.

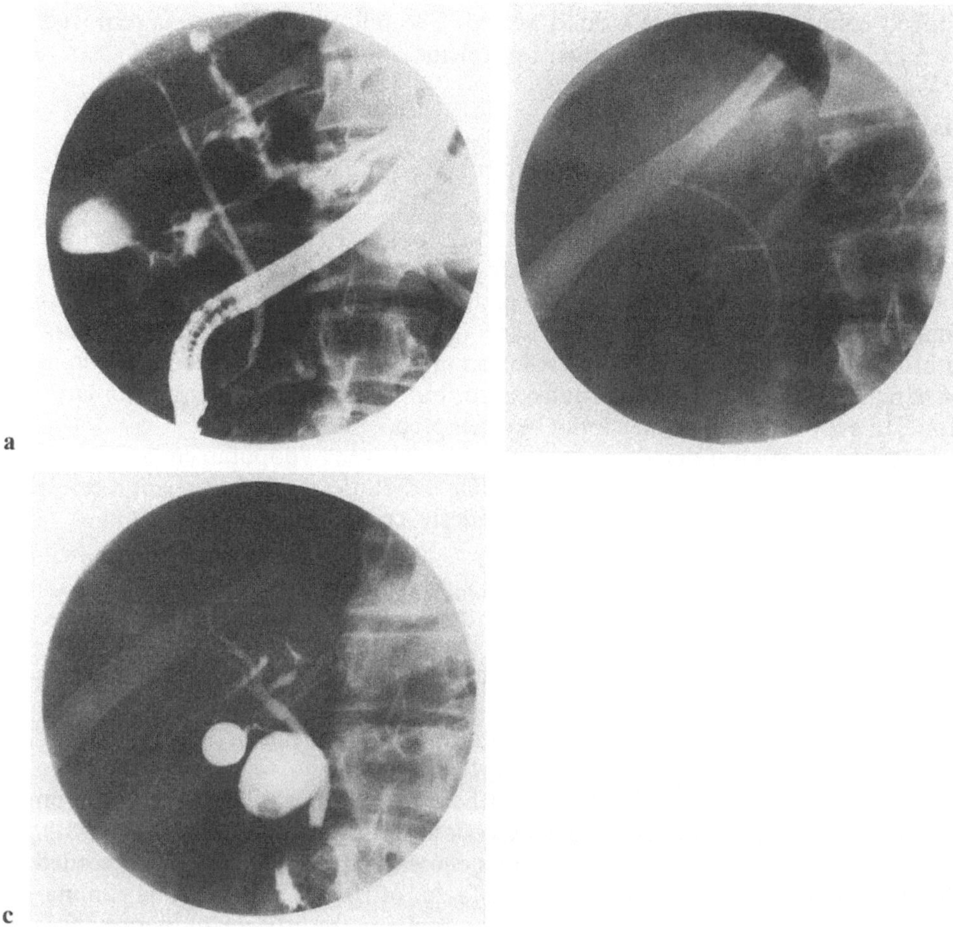


**Fig. 3. a** Endoscopic retrograde cholangiography demonstrates the laceration of the left hepatic duct and the large extravasation of the contrast medium. **b** Bilionasal drain in situ. Native X-ray film with subject in supine position. The tube has the same position as in Fig. 2 with its tip at the hepatic junction. **c** The tube has been extracted after its final use for a retrograde cholangiogram 3 weeks after the insertion. There only remains a very small extravasation beside the left hepatic duct. It is not possible to determine whether the periphery of the left lobe is well drained or not

## Treatment of a Bilicutaneous Fistula

Bilicutaneous fistulas are normally treated by surgery, however, the nasobiliary drain may also be useful here. A 28-year-old man from our series of patients, for example, was suffering from a stab wound of the abdomen. A laceration of the liver was surgically closed. Some days later, large amounts of bile began flowing from the drain into the wound. Leakage of the left hepatic duct was demonstrated by endoscopic retrograde cholangiography (Fig. 3). After insertion of a bilionasal tube and application of low-pressure suction, the bile flow from the drain stopped completely, and the wound healed. The bilionasal drain was removed 2 weeks later without any subsequent problems.

### Dissolution of Common Duct Stones

Residual bile duct stones may be dissolved via a T-tube (Leuschner et al. 1981). The use of the bilionasal tube makes it possible to dissolve bile duct stones without prior surgery using our schedule (Leuschner et al. 1981) of alternate flushing with a glyceryl 1-mono-octanoate preparation for cholesterol dissolution and a bile acid-ethylenediaminetetraacetate solution to dissolve calcium bilirubinate. Our success rate is about 66% (of 42 patients there was complete dissolution in 16 patients, incomplete dissolution in 12 patients, and no dissolution in 14 patients). This is not exceptionally good, but in high-risk patients with large stones this low-risk treatment should be attempted.

Side effects, such as diarrhea, nausea, pain, and even hypopotassemia are common. The importance of this method of stone dissolution is decreasing as a result of the new techniques for mechanical stone destruction.

### Aspiration of Bile for Chemical and Bacteriological Tests

Bile may be aspired through the nasobiliary tube at any time. To obtain bile showing the actual degree of bacterial colonization, it is necessary to discard an initially aspirated volume equal to two to three times the capacity of the tube (i.e., 2–5 ml). We found a constant level of bacterial colonization of the bile in the study of several controls.

Using this technique of nasobiliary catheterization in patients with common duct stones, we measured the biliary excretion of mezlocillin (Helm et al. 1981). Remarkably, this is reduced in cholangitis/cholestasis, but nevertheless exceeded the minimal inhibitory concentration by a factor of 10–100. The bacteria elimination rate from the bile, a new parameter for studying the efficacy of therapy, was even reduced in these cases. The direct access to the bile duct also permits continuous study of bile composition for several days under varying conditions. There is, for example, a persisting diurnal rhythm of cholesterol saturation of the bile after cholecystectomy and papillotomy (Kurtz et al. 1982). However, the concentration of bile acid at the same time remains constant.

### Drainage in Malignant Obstruction of the Common Bile Duct

Biliary drainage in obstruction by a tumor may be accomplished externally by the percutaneous transhepatic technique or by means of the bilionasal tube. These methods lead to a bile-loss syndrome. Biliary-duodenal stents are internal drains which have the advantage of a more normal flow of bile. Internal drainage (pig tail or stents), the more physiological approach, should be done whenever possible. Most tumors that obstruct the bile ducts can not be resected. In such cases, internal drainage via biliary-duodenal stents has proven to be an excellent palliative procedure with low risk and high efficacy. External drainages should only be done if an operation is planned, as a definitive palliative procedure in patients with severe complaints as a result of cholestasis, especially permanent itching, or if internal drainage is not possible.

## Summary and Conclusions

The endoscopically introduced self-fixing bilionasal drain has been thoroughly evaluated and the technique for its use is fully developed. Its main therapeutic value is in acute obstructive suppurative cholangitis. The second practical application is the prevention of stone impaction after endoscopic papillotomy. The study of bacterial elimination kinetics in relation to antibiotic therapy is a new method to investigate the efficacy of antibiotics. This is still an investigative technique with theoretical aspects and practical consequences. Control of the chemical composition of the bile until now has been a theoretical concept.

## References

Classen M, Geenen J, Kawai K (1979) The papilla Vateri and its diseases – International workshop. Witzstrock, Baden-Baden

Cotton PB, Barney PGJ, Mason RR (1979) Transnasal bile duct catheterization after endoscopic sphincterotomy. Gut 20:285–287

Helm EB, Wurbs D, Gundlach H, Beyer B, Hagenmüller F, Stille W (1981) Keimelimination und Konzentrationsbestimmungen unter Mezlocillin in der Galle bei Gallenwegsinfektionen. Dtsch Med Wochenschr 106:1087–1090

Kurtz W, Leuschner U, Schneider S, Phillip J, Hagenmüller F, Wurbs D, Classen M (1982) Fortbestehende diurnale Rhythmi, der biliären Cholesterinsättigung nach Cholezystektomie und Papillotomie. Z Gastroenterol 20:541–542

Leuschner U, Wurbs D, Baumgärtel H, Helm E, Classen M (1981) Alternating treatment of common bile duct stones with a modified glyceril-1-monooctanoate preparation and a bile acid EDTA solution by nasobiliary tube. Scand Gastroenterol 16:497–503

Nagai N, Toki F, Oi J, Suzuki H, Kozu T, Taker T (1976) Continuous endoscopic pancreato-choledochal catheterization. Gastrointest Endosc 23:78–81

Schoenfield LJ (1971) Biliary excretion of antibiotics. N Engl J Med 284:1213–1214 (editorial)

Shapiro HA, Cotton PB (1975) Leaving a balloon tip catheter in the bile duct at duodenoscopy. Lancet II:13–14

Wurbs D, Classen M (1977) Transpapillary longstanding tube for hepatobiliary drainage. Endoscopy 9:192–193

Wurbs D (1982) Endoscopic papillotomy. Scand J Gastroenterol [Suppl] 77:107–115

# 14 Chemical Treatment of Choledocholithiasis

*U. Leuschner, H. Baumgärtel, and J. Klempa*

## Treatment of Choledocholithiasis

The first attempt at bile duct stone dissolution took place in 1892. But it is only in the last decade that new perfusion media have been developed.

## Dissolution Media

A 4.3% cholate solution was used for cholesterol bile duct stone dissolution (Lansford et al. 1974; Iser et al. 1976). Intrahepatic stones were treated with a 0.34% chenodeoxycholic acid solution (Czygan et al. 1977). In 1978 glyceryl-1-monooctanoin (Capmul 8210) was introduced, which dissolves stones 2.5 times faster than bile salt solutions (Thistle et al. 1980). Bile salt solutions and monooctanoin only dissolve cholesterol stones. Since recurrent stones after cholecystectomy consist up to 40% of calcium bilirubinate (Schenk et al. 1979 a) we have developed a bile salt-EDTA solution that will also be effective for calcium-biliru-

**Table 1.** Dissolution media for retained bile duct stones

| | |
|---|---|
| a) Cholate–Na | 4.3% |
| b) Chenodeoxycholate–Na | 0.345% |
| c) Capmul 8210 | |
| Glyceril-1-monooctanoate | 70% |
| Glyceril dioctanoate | 30% |
| Glyceril trioctanoate | |
| Caprylic acid | |
| d) GMOC | |
| Glyceril-1-monooctanoate | 93% |
| Pluronic F 68 } stabilizer | 2.5%-3.6% |
| Palmidrol } stabilizer | 0.3%-0.6% |
| Cholic acid | 0.4% |
| Water | |
| e) BA–EDTA (pH 9.4) | |
| Ursodeoxycholic acid | 0.5% |
| Cholic acid | 0.5% |
| EDTA-2Na | 1.0% |
| Carnosine | 0.3% |
| Water | |

Infusion speed: a, b, and e, 20–30 ml/h; c and d, 2–6 ml/h
Infusion pressure: 20–30 cm $H_2O$

binate stones (Leuschner and Baumgärtel 1982). EDTA binds calcium, the binding capacity becoming more effective the further the pH is shifted into the alkaline range. As in the in vivo situation it is not known before the onset of treatment whether we are dealing with a radiolucent composition stone containing cholesterol and pigments or with a calcium-bilirubinate stone with a minor cholesterol content, we use the BA-EDTA solution alternately with a special preparation of Capmul 8210 (GMOC) (Leuschner et al. 1982). Thus we try to extract the cholesterol and the calcium fraction from the stones, which induces disaggregation of the concrement (Table 1).

The effect of this treatment has been demonstrated in several in vitro investigations (Leuschner et al. 1980). The stones had dissolved 30–80 h after the alternating treatment. The same effect has been seen in bovine bilirubinate stones.

## Indications

An inquiry directed at 46 gastroenterology units yielded data from 16 units (Table 2).

Concerning the administration of perfusion therapy the inquiry revealed the following results: In the simultaneous presence of gallbladder and bile duct stones perfusion therapy is only performed if stones have failed to be removed by either surgery or endoscopic stone extraction. Only in two centers was endoscopic stone extraction of bile duct stones given priority over surgery.

In the presence of a T tube in 9 of 16 units stone extraction is tried first, in 5 of 16 units perfusion is first attempted, and in two units the staff tend to perform surgery if extraction has failed.

If the T tube has been removed, 11 units will start with stone extraction and attempt dissolution subsequently, while 5 units favour reoperation after failed extraction.

This means that the longer the interval after cholecystectomy becomes, the more conservative the procedures will be; obviously endoscopic stone extraction is the first attempt before dissolution therapy in most units.

## Results

Table 3 shows the results of the inquiry and results from the literature, as far as overlapping could be excluded for sure. In 129 patients treated with cholate or chenodeoxycholate partial or complete success was achieved in 54%. The results quoted in the literature are obviously more favourable than those of the inquiry, where success was only achieved in a total of 40%.

With Capmul therapy the inquiry revealed a total success rate of 40% in 110 patients. The inquiry of Alan Hofmann in 270 patients revealed the same result. The result quoted in the literature, 65%, is again more favourable. With a total of 475 patients a mean success rate of 48% was found (Table 4).

Data on alternating treatment with GMOC and BA-EDTA are still scarce. The inquiry revealed an overall success rate of 76%, against 61% in our own collective. The alternating treatment seems to provide better results than therapy with other dissolving agents, with a mean rate of 68%, but the number of patients treated is small (Table 5).

**Table 2.** Sources of data

| |
|---|
| Caspary, W.: Hanau, W. Germany |
| Cotton, P. B.: London, Great Britain |
| Czygan, P.: Heidelberg, W. Germany |
| Federlin, K.: Giessen, W. Germany |
| Geenen, J. E.: Racine, USA |
| Hofmann, A. F.: San Diego, USA[a] |
| Koch, H.: Schweinfurt, W. Germany |
| Lesterhuis, W., Tytgat, G. N.: Amsterdam, Netherlands |
| Manegold, B. C.: Mannheim, W. Germany |
| Paumgartner, G.: Munich, W. Germany |
| Rösch, W. Frankfurt/M, W. Germany |
| Safrany, L.: Wilhelmshaven, W. Germany |
| Schmack, B.: Erlangen, W. Germany |
| Seifert, E.: Koblenz, W. Germany |
| Terblanche, J.: Cape Town, South Africa |
| Thistle, J. L.: Rochester, USA |
| Tweedle, D.: Manchester, Great Britain |

[a] See table 4

**Table 3.** Dissolution of bile duct stones with cholate or chenodeoxycholate

| | No. of pts | Mean age (years) | Dosage (ml/h) | Success | Partial success | Treatment time (days) |
|---|---|---|---|---|---|---|
| Inquiry (1982) | | | | | | |
| Cholate | 26 | 65 | 10–15 | 8 (31%) | 2 (8%) | 11 |
| Cheno | 5 | 65 | 2–5 | 2 | 0 | 10 (–25 weeks) |
| Literature (1973–1981) | | | | | | |
| Cholate | 98 | | 10–15 | 58 (59%) | | |
| Total | 129 | 65 | | 70 (54%) | | |

**Table 4.** Dissolution of bile duct stones with Capmul 8210

| | No. of pts | Mean age (years) | Dosage (ml/h) | Success | Partial success | Treatment time (days) |
|---|---|---|---|---|---|---|
| Inquiry (1982) | 110 | 64 | 1–15 | 22 (20%) | 22 (20%) | 10 |
| Inquiry (1982) A. F. Hofmann | 270 | | | 90 (33%) | 30 (11%) | |
| Literature (1978–1981) | 95 | | | 62 (65%) | | |
| Total | 475 | | | 226 (48%) | | |

Nevertheless, exact comparison of the individual dissolving agents is impossible. Data reported in the literature are too sparse. Thus, for example, data on the mode of administration, duration of therapy, and especially stone size were often not given. Therefore we decided not to intensify our inquiry, not least in view of the experience that the recovery rate of questionaires is in reverse proportion to their volume.

**Table 5.** Dissolution of bile duct stones with GMOC/BA–EDTA

| | No. of pts | Mean age (years) | Dosage (ml/h) | Success | Partial success | Treatment time (days) |
|---|---|---|---|---|---|---|
| Inquiry (1982) | 30 | 64 | 2–6/20 | 10 (33%) | 13 (43%) | 6 (–236) |
| own data (1981–1982) | 44 | 73 | 5/20 | 27 (61%) | | 19 |
| Total | 74 | 68 | | 50 (68%) | | 12 |

**Table 6.** Side-effects of dissolution therapy in bile duct stone patients (data from 16 gastroenterological units)

| | Cholangitis | Pancreatitis | Ulcers | Fatalities | Other |
|---|---|---|---|---|---|
| Cholate | 4/26 (15%) | – | – | 2/26 | 20/26 |
| Cheno | – | – | – | – | 3/5 |
| Capmul 8210 | 8/110 (7%) | – | 2/110 | – | 86/110 |
| GMOC/ BA–EDTA | 1/74 (1%) | – | – | – | 52/74 |

The tangible results of our investigation are an overall success rate of approx. 50%; the combined use of a lipid solubilizer and a bile salt-EDTA solution could open new prospects and up to now perfusion therapy has been performed in only 700 patients. This makes up clear that it is no alternative to endoscopic stone extraction, but a complementary method.

Side-effects are summarized in Table 6. Vomiting, diarrhea and abdominal cramps occur with all agents in 60%–80% of cases. Cholangitis seems to be rather rare; in two patients receiving Capmul duodenal ulcers were seen.

## Toxicity in Animal Experiments and Man

In 1977 Mack et al. reported that 4 of 5 Rhesus monkeys receiving cholate infusions had died. Severe inflammation of the biliary tree was noted. With Capmul 8210 only mild alterations were detectable (Mack et al. 1978). In 1979 Schenk (Schenk et al. 1979b) found severe, partly hemorrhagic inflammation in 17 cats and in 1981 Götz observed similar alterations in rats (Götz et al. 1981) after similar medication.

In our own investigations (unpublished data) we have treated female Wistar rats for 10 h and for 7 and 11 days with GMOC and BA-EDTA via esophageal tube. The histological examination of all organs showed no pathological findings. Ten mongrel dogs received cholate, chenodeoxycholate, Capmul 8210, GMOC, BA-EDTA, and physiological saline solution as a constant infusion via the bile fistula over 50 h. Cholate induced severe hemorrhagic inflammation; less intensive alterations were seen with Capmul and GMOC; still less pronounced changes with chenodeoxycholate and BA-EDTA; and no changes with saline solution. Extensive biochemical investigations will be reported elsewhere.

Histological investigations of patients have proved rather difficult. In two patients receiving Capmul 8210 duodenal erosions were seen (Schenk et al. 1980). In four of our own patients treated with GMOC and BA-EDTA histological alterations of the biliary tree could not be unequivocally differentiated from changes that occur in untreated patients suffering from bile duct stones. While serum levels of calcium and copper stayed unchanged in patients treated for 10 days, there was a significant fall in the zinc level, an aspect to be considered in the future.

## Conclusions

Dissolution therapy of bile duct stones is successful in approx. 50% of cases. This therapy is usually performed after failure of endoscopic stone extraction. All known dissolution agents induce considerable local side-effects in animal experiments; side-effects seem to be milder in man, but the indications for perfusion therapy should be strictly limited.

## References


Czygan P, Stiehl A, Fröhling W, Kommerell B, Encke A (1977) Therapie intrahepatischer Cholesterinsteine durch Chenodesoxycholsäure. Dtsch Med Wschr 102:518–520

Götz R, Raedsch R, Waldherr R, Walker S, Stiehl A, Kommerell B (1981) Lokal toxische Wirkung von Glyceriloctanoat-Präparationen. Z. Gastroenterol 19:549–550

Iser JH, Saxton H, Wiegard J, Dowling RH (1976) Efficacy and complications of T-tube cholate infusion in the treatment of retained common bile duct (CBD) stones. Gut 17:815–816

Lansford C, Mehta S, Kern F (1974) The treatment of retained stones in the common bile duct with sodium cholate infusion. Gut 15:48–51

Leuschner U, Baumgärtel H, Wurbs D (1980) Dissolution of cholesterol bile duct stones with a modified Capmul 8210-emulsion and with an EDTA solution. Leber Magen Darm 10:284–287

Leuschner U, Baumgärtel H (1982) Gallstone dissolution in the biliary tract: in vitro investigations on inhibiting factors and special dissolution agents. Am J Gastroenterol 77:222–226

Leuschner U, Baumgärtel H, Phillip J, Jessen K, Hagenmüller F, Trüber E, Classen M (1982) Combined irrigation and endoscopy in the treatment of biliary duct stones. Dtsch Med Wschr 107:285–290

Mack E, Saito Ch, Goldfarb St, Carlson GL, Hofmann AF (1977) Local toxicity of T-tube-infused cholate in the rhesus monkey. Surg Forum 28:408–409

Mack EA, Saito CH, Goldfarb St, Crummy A, Thistle JL, Carlson GL, Babayan VK, Hofmann AF (1978) A new agent for gallstone dissolution: experimental and clinical evaluation. Surg Forum 29:438–439

Schenk J, Wosiewitz U, Rösch W, Schmack B (1979a) Untersuchungen zur Genese von Choledochus-Rezidivsteinen nach Cholezystektomie. Z Gastroenterol 9:645–646

Schenk J, Koch H, Stolte M, Schmack B (1979b) Tissue compatibility of the gallstone solubilizer Capmul 8210 – a study in cats. Gastroenterology 76:1237 A

Schenk J, Schmack B, Rösch W, Riemann JF, Koch H, Demling L (1980) Spülbehandlung von Choledochussteinen mit Octanoat (Capmul 8210). Dtsch Med Wschr 105:917–921

Thistle JL, Carlson GL, Hofmann AF, La Russo NF, MacCarty RL, Flynn GL, Higuchi WI, Babayan VK (1980) Monooctanoin, a dissolution agent for retained cholesterol bile duct stones. Physical properties and clinical application. Gastroenterology 78:1016–1022

# 15 Endoscopic Implantation of Biliodudenal Endoprostheses in Benign Bile Duct Stenoses

*N. Soehendra, K. de Heer, and J. Kempeneers*

Benign stenoses of the choledochus are usually a rare indication for drainage.

The following constricting diseases in the region of the common bile duct may be considered to indicate drainage when causal therapy can no longer be considered:

Unextractable choledochus stones
Postoperative stricture
Chronic pancreatitis
Sclerosing cholangitis
Biliary fistula.

## Unextractable Choledochus Stones

Stones in the common bile duct can mostly be removed either by surgery or by means of endoscopy. Endoscopic papillotomy is usually the only choice in inoperable patients. With the Dormia basket 85%–90% of stones can be extracted. In recent years attempts have been made to crush very large stones in the choledochus. Nevertheless some choledochus stones cannot be extracted. If they cause jaundice a transpapillary endoprosthesis can be implanted as a palliative measure (Fig. 1). If bacterial cholangitis is present at the same time a nasobiliary tube for antibiotic rinsing should first be introduced (Fig. 2).

## Postoperative Stricture

Postoperative strictures are a rare complication of bile duct surgery. Mostly they result from injuries in the area of the middle main bile duct or from disturbances following T-tube drainage (Fig. 3).

Such strictures are frequently manifest and must therefore be removed. Correction is carried out surgically, mostly by means of a biliodigestive anastomosis. An endoscopic dilatation with a balloon catheter can be tried in small strictures that are not too narrow. For long, high-grade strictures in patients who are inoperable because of some other disease or advanced age, the transpapillary endoprosthesis is useful as a palliative method.

## Chronic Pancreatitis

One of the most common complications of advanced sclerosing pancreatitis is stenosis of the distal choledochus. If treatment becomes necessary the usual pro-

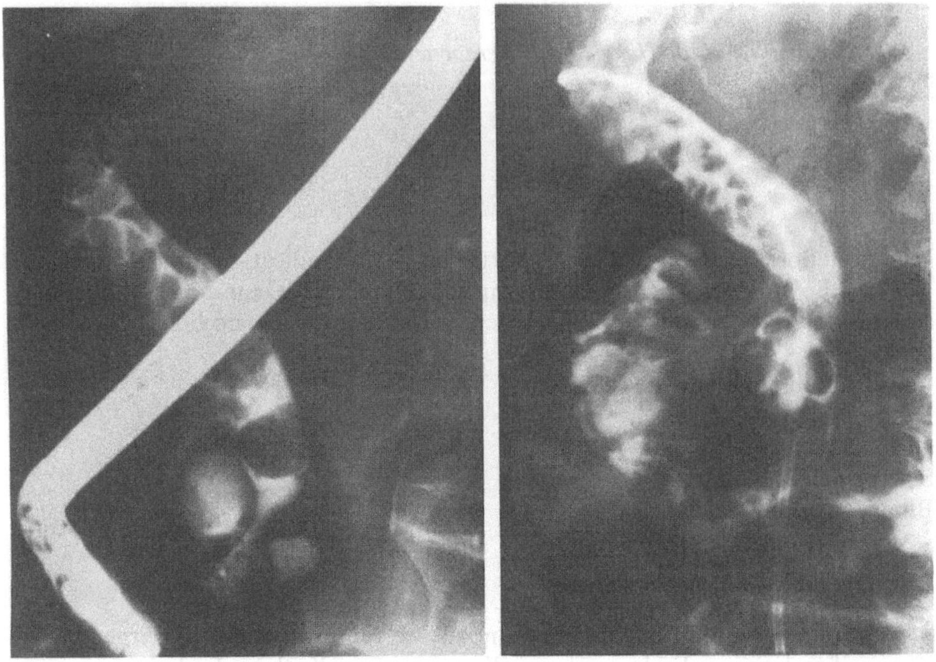

**Fig. 1.** Surgically and endoscopically unremovable choledochus stones with obstructive jaundice. Palliative transpapillary drainage with a pigtail catheter. (W. Cook, Denmark)

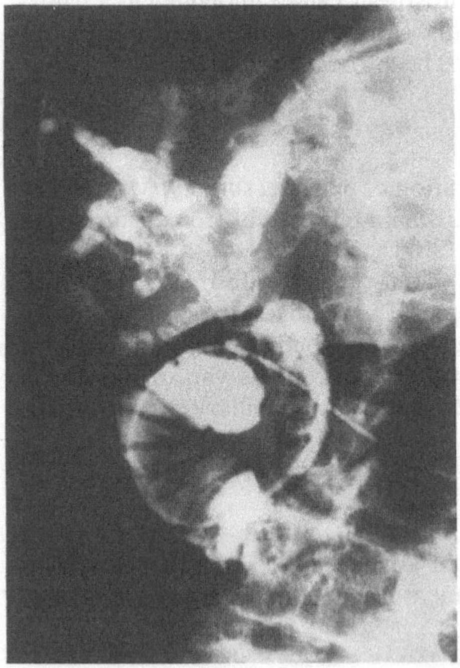

**Fig. 2.** Stone impaction with bacterial cholangitis. Immediate treatment with nasobiliary tube. (W. Cook, Denmark)

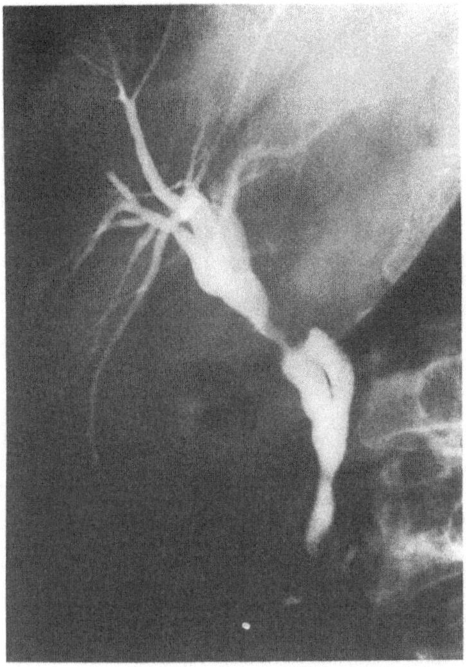

**Fig. 3.** Postoperative stricture after surgical T-tube drainage

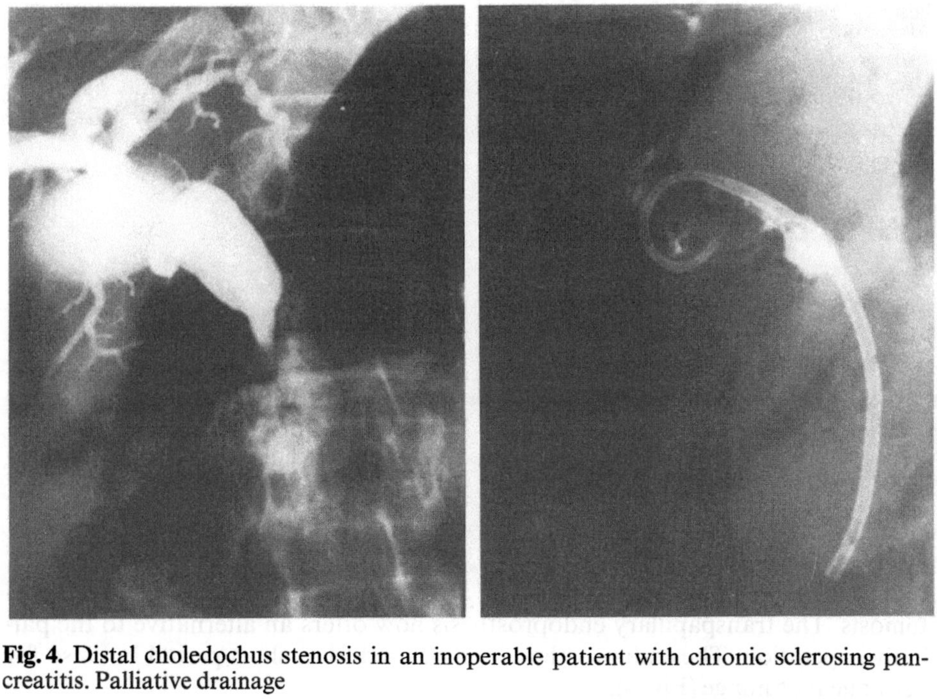

**Fig. 4.** Distal choledochus stenosis in an inoperable patient with chronic sclerosing pancreatitis. Palliative drainage

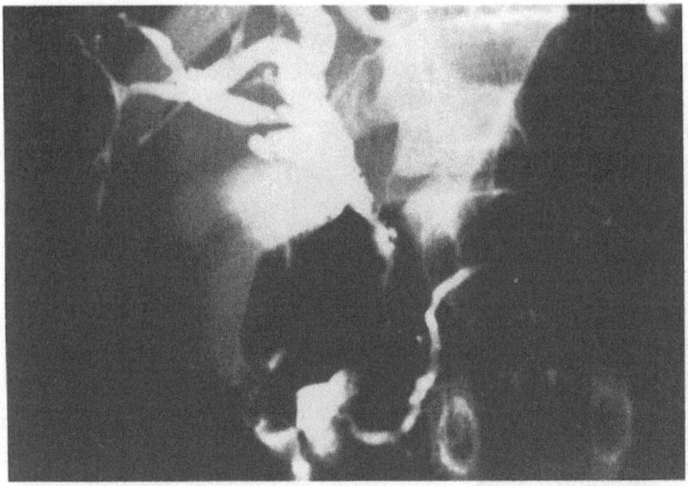

**Fig. 5.** Sclerosing cholangitis: an indication for transpapillary drainage

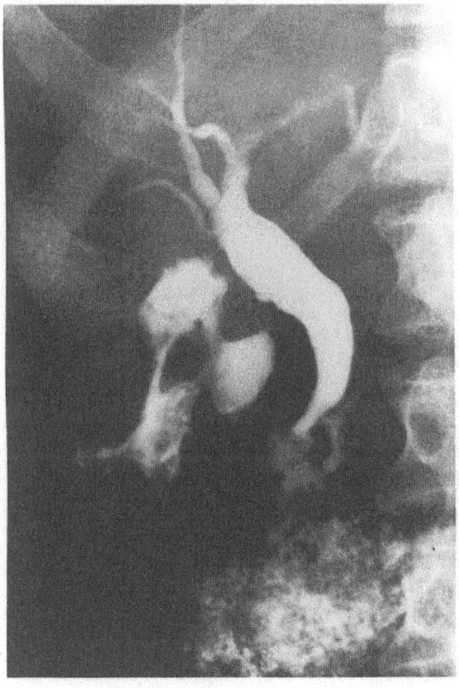

**Fig. 6.** Inadequate suturing of the cystic stump after cholecystectomy necessitated by a bile outflow disturbance

cedure is the Whipple operation or, as a palliative method, biliodigestive anastomosis. The transpapillary endoprosthesis now offers an alternative to the palliative operation. The endoprosthesis can be used for a short period but also for permanent drainage (Fig. 4).

## Sclerosing Cholangitis

The etiology of primary sclerosing cholangitis is still unknown, and to date only symptomatic treatment is possible. Removal of the high-grade obstructions of the bile ducts is at the center of therapeutic efforts. Endless and percutaneous transhepatic drainages have been used so far. The endoscopic drainage is a further method (Fig. 5).

## Biliary fistula

Postoperative biliary fistulas usually close up by themselves, provided the bile flow is not disturbed. Frequent causes are the unremarked cutting of bile ducts and inadequate suturing of the stump of the cystic duct (Fig. 6). There is no urgency if adequate drainage is possible. Reversible drainage problems in the distal choledochus or in the papilla of Vater can be corrected easily and with no great problems with an endoprosthesis until the fistula has closed.

The transpapillary introduction of an endoprosthesis is a new method (Soehendra and Reynders-Frederix 1979). Its use in benign strictures has been much rarer

**Table 1.** Total numbers of transpapillary endoprostheses inserted in benign stenosis at 13 centers

| Endoscopist | *n* |
|---|---|
| Cotton, England | 8 |
| Geenen, USA | 12 |
| Hagenmüller, Classen, W. Germany | 6 |
| Huibregtse, Tytgat, Holland | 20 |
| v. Husen, W. Germany | 0 |
| Kühner, Stölzle, Ottenjann, W. Germany | 26 |
| Liguory, France | 0 |
| Manegold, W. Germany | 0 |
| Riemann, Demling, W. Germany | 2 |
| Seifert, W. Germany | 0 |
| Soehendra, W. Germany | 12 |
| Schott, Safrany, W. Germany | 5 |
| Wurbs, W. Germany | 6 |

**Table 2.** Transpapillary endoprosthesis in benign stenosis: Indications and success rate

| Indication | Attempted | Failed |
|---|---|---|
| Unextractable stones | 53 | – |
| Postoperative stricture | 18 | 2 |
| Chronic pancreatitis | 10 | – |
| Sclerosing cholangitis | 10 | 3 |
| Biliary fistula | 4 | – |
| Other | 2 | – |
| | 97 (=100%) | 5 (=5.2%) |

**Table 3.** Complications of transpapillary endoprosthesis in benign stenosis

| Complication | *n* | % |
|---|---|---|
| Obstruction without cholangitis | 6 | 6.2 |
| Obstruction with cholangitis | 3 | 3.1 |
| Dislodgement | 1 | 1.0 |

Complication rate 10.3%; no mortality

than in malignant tumors. We have made enquiries of endoscopic centers around the world to gain more information about it. Of 16 centers approached, 13 responded. In 4 of them benign stenosis of the choledochus is not seen as an indication for drainage. In the remaining 9 hospitals transpapillary drainage has been applied in benign strictures a total of 97 times (Table 1). The patients were 62 women and 35 men aged 26 to 94 years, the average age being 69 years. The success rate of the method was 95%. Compared with the results in malignant tumors this is 5%–10% higher (Huibregtse 1981; Soehendra et al. 1982). Failures were registered in the use of the drainage for postoperative strictures and sclerosing cholangitis. In other uncomplicated stenoses the method was always successful. The main indication is unextractable choledochus stones (Table 2).

The complication rate was 10.3%, no lethality being registered. The most common complication was obstruction of the catheter, resulting in cholangitis. Dislocation of the prosthesis was observed in one case. There was no need for surgical correction in any case with complications. They were all treated by changing the catheter endoscopically (Table 3).

According to the experience collected, there is a legitimate indication for the use of a transpapillary endoprosthesis in benign stenosis. It is a palliative procedure to allow drainage when causal therapy no longer is possible or seems to involve too high a risk for the patient. This method is usually used for long-term drainage, but can also be used instead of the nasobiliary tube for temporary pur-

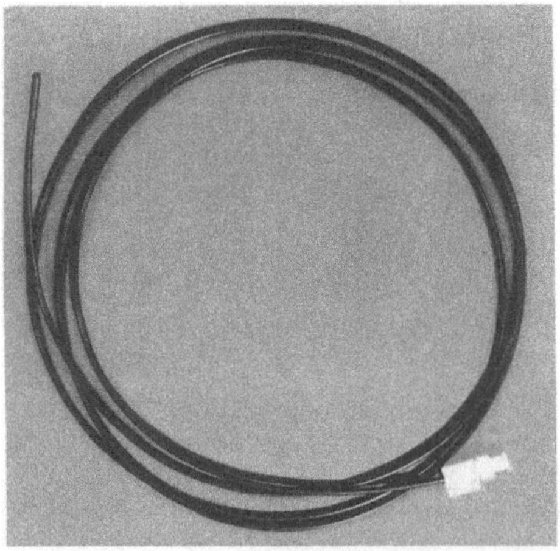

**Fig. 7.** Tapered special catheter for cannulation of long high-grade strictures. (W. Cook, Denmark)

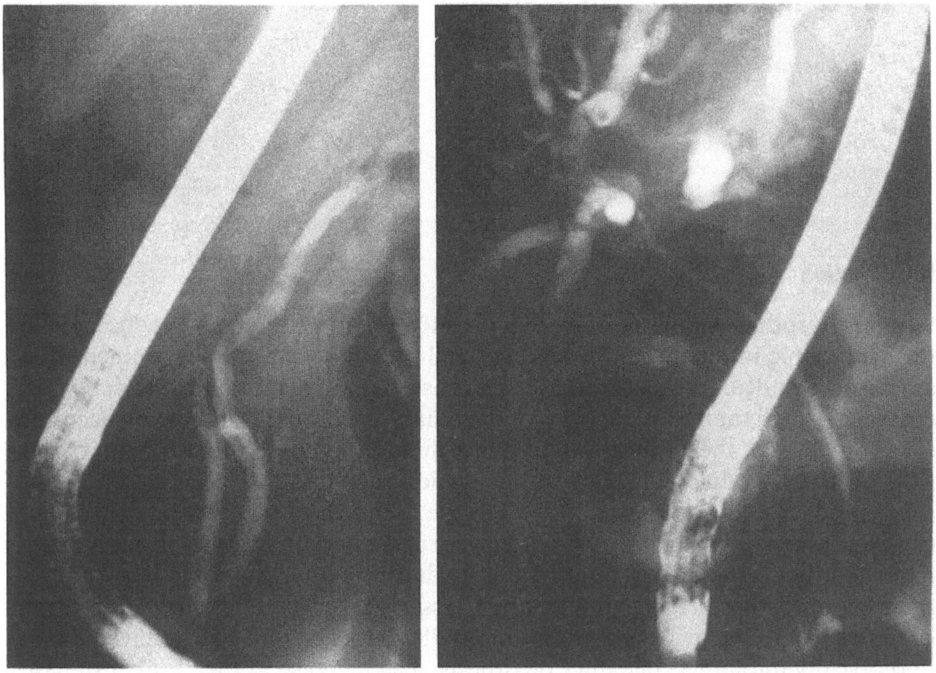

**Fig. 8.** Complete cholangiography using the tapered catheter in a case with obstructed choledochus

poses. Unlike the nasobiliary tube the endoprosthesis does not cause a bile-loss syndrome and is not uncomfortable for the patient.

The complications observed to date have not been severe and can be corrected by means of endoscopy. Therefore this procedure seems to be a low-risk therapy for benign stenosis. The procedure is usually easy in uncomplicated strictures. It is not always necessary to perform papillotomy first. In long, high-grade strictures insertion of the prosthesis may become difficult. For such cases we recommend the use of a special catheter (Fig. 7). This catheter is 170 cm long and 7 Fr. thick, with a tapered tip; it allows insertion of the guide wire through long, high-graded strictures because the wire can be twisted in any direction. With this drilling technique complete choledochus strictures can sometimes be recanalized. For orientation it is possible to use the catheter for cholangiography. Afterwards this special catheter is used for dilatation to ease the insertion of the prosthesis (Fig. 8).

## References


Huibregtse K et al. (1981) Transpapillary positioning of a large 3.2 mm biliary endoprosthesis. Endoscopy 13:217–219

Soehendra N, Reynders-Frederix V (1979) Palliative Gallengangdrainage. Dtsch Med Wschr 104:206–207

Soehendra N et al. (1982) Transpapilläre Endoprothese. In: Endoskopische Prothetik. Acron, Berlin

# 16 Results of Endoscopic Bilioduodenal Drainage in Malignant Bile Duct Stenoses

*F. Hagenmüller*

## Introduction

Since its introduction in the year 1979 (Soehendra and Reynders-Frederix 1979), the endoscopic implantation of biliduodenal prostheses has rapidly gained widespread acceptance. Its most common use is as a palliative measure to effect biliary drainage in malignant obstructions of the biliary system. This indication accounts for about 86% of the applications of this technique, as compared with biliary outflow obstruction due to benign causes, which accounts for the remaining 14% (Hagenmüller and Soehendra 1983). On the occasion of a conference on biliary drainage procedures held in 1981, data were presented on 89 patients with malignant stenosis of the biliary tract treated palliatively by endoscopic implantation of an endoprosthesis (Hagenmüller and Classen 1982). A worldwide study carried out in May 1982 provides information on 380 patients who had received an endoscopically implanted bile duct prosthesis. The increase in the number of cases reflects the rapid spread of the procedure.

In the present paper the results of these collective statistics are discussed together with the results obtained in our own patients.

## Material and Methods

In May 1982, six European endoscopists with particular experience in the use of biliary drainage procedures were requested to provide information on the results they had achieved with endoscopically implanted biliduodenal endoprosthesis in patients presenting with malignant obstruction of the biliary passage. The request was addressed to the following endoscopists: P. B. Cotton, London; K. Huibregtse, Amsterdam; L. Safrany, Wilhelmshaven; N. Soehendra, Hamburg; D. Wurbs, Hamburg; as well as to our own department (M. Classen, F. Hagenmüller). A questionnaire was employed in the collection of data on the number of patients, indications, technique, complications, and clinical course. In addition, we analyzed our own patients who received a biliduodenal endoprosthesis in the period between May 1979 and March 1982. In the patients of this group who died, the following parameters were investigated for possible influence on the survival times: age of the patient, serum albumin and bilirubin concentrations prior to endoprosthesis implantation, the decrease in serum bilirubin concentration following implantation, the presence of metastases, and the localization of the bile duct stenosis.

**Results and Discussion**

All the investigators approached responded to the enquiry and together provided data on a total of 454 patients in whom endoscopic implantation of a biliduodenal endoprosthesis had been indicated to treat malignant obstruction of bile outflow.

*Technique.* All the participating endoscopists regularly use the same implantation technique, which is that originally described by Soehendra and Reynders-Frederix (1979). First, an endoscopic retrograde cholangiopancreatography is performed, the aim of which is to provide information on the anatomy of the biliary ducts and to confirm the indication. The endoprosthesis employed is made of polytetrafluorethylene (Teflon), polyethylene, or polyurethane. The individual endoscopists have their own preferences with respect to the design and material of the endoprosthesis employed (see Fig. 1 and Sect. 12 Technique). The length of the endoprosthesis is determined by the individual anatomical situation. All the participants in the study perform a small prior endoscopic papillotomy, which facilitates the insertion of the endoprosthesis into the common bile duct. The duct is sounded with the aid of a guide wire, over which the prosthesis is fitted and then inserted with the aid of a "pusher" (introducer) tube until it reaches the desired position within the bile duct. Thereafter, the introducer tube, guide wire, and endoscope are removed (Fig. 2).

Since April 1981, all the participating endoscopists have been using only a lateral-viewing endoscope provided with an instrument channel having a diameter

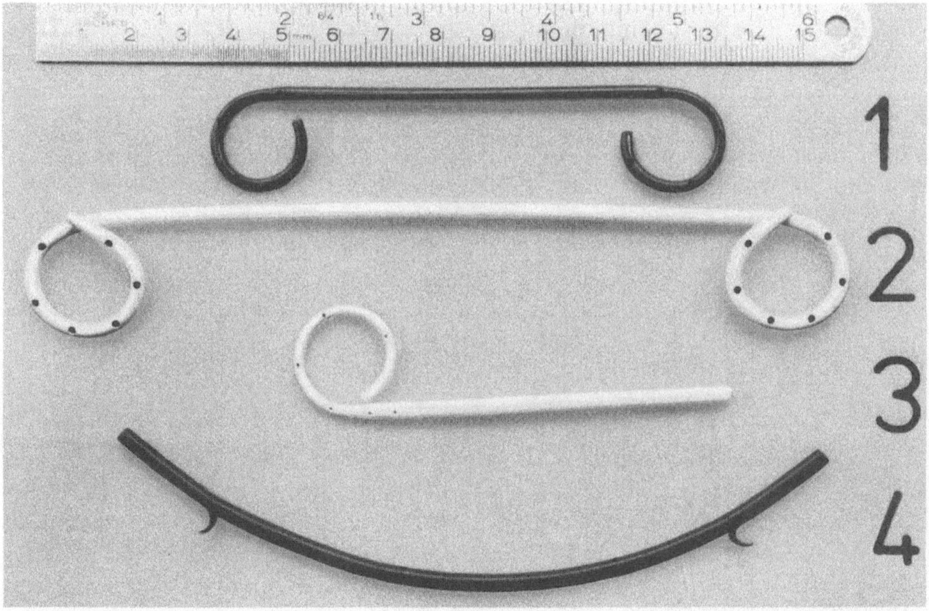


**Fig. 1.** Biliduodenal endoprostheses with an outer diameter of 3.3 mm (10 French) for endosopic implantation. *1*, Double-pigtail polytetrafluorethylene (Teflon) endoprosthesis; *2*, double-pigtail polyurethane endoprosthesis; *3*, mono-pigtail polyethylene endoprosthesis; *4*, straight polyethylene endoprosthesis with side flaps

of 3.7 mm (Fig. 3) (Hagenmüller and Classen 1982). Using this endoscope, it is possible to place an endoprosthesis having an outside diameter of 3.3 mm (10 French). Endoprostheses with outside diameters of 5 and 7 French are considered by all the endoscopists to be inadequate, since they become blocked relatively quickly by "sludge" and thus become nonfunctional. In contrast to the choice of material for the prosthesis, the technical aspects of the procedure of endoscopic endoprosthesis implantation are standardized.

A *technical variant* is the placement of an endoprosthesis in both the right and left hepatic ducts. This is desirable when a stenosis of the bifurcation of the common hepatic duct interrupts the communication between the ducts draining the right and left lobes of the liver, so that the two lobes need to be drained selectively (Fig. 4). The combination of the endoscopic implantation technique with the percutaneous-transhepatic procedure can also be useful when either technique alone is unable to achieve satisfactory drainage (Fig. 5).

Of a total of 454 patients, endoscopic implantation of an endoprosthesis was successful in 380 cases. Thus, the technical success rate of the procedure was 83.7%. The most frequent cause of a technical failure of the procedure was the inaccessibility of Vater's papilla, for example in patients with duodenal stenosis or prior gastric resection. In such cases, the endoprosthesis must be implanted via the percutaneous-transhepatic route. When the endoscopic and percutaneous-transhepatic approaches are employed as complementary procedures, the implantation of the endoprosthesis is successful in almost 100% of cases.

*Indications.* The most common indication for biliduodenal drainage, at 45.7% of cases, proved to be carcinoma of the pancreas (Table 1). The second most common indication was bile duct carcinoma (18.4% of cases), followed by carcinoma

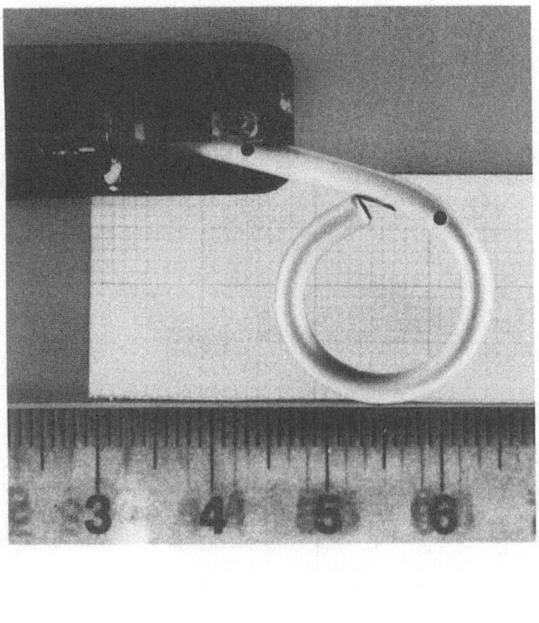


**Fig. 3.** Distal tip of the side-viewing duodenoscope "Olympus JF-1T 3.7 mm" loaded with a 10-French endoprosthesis

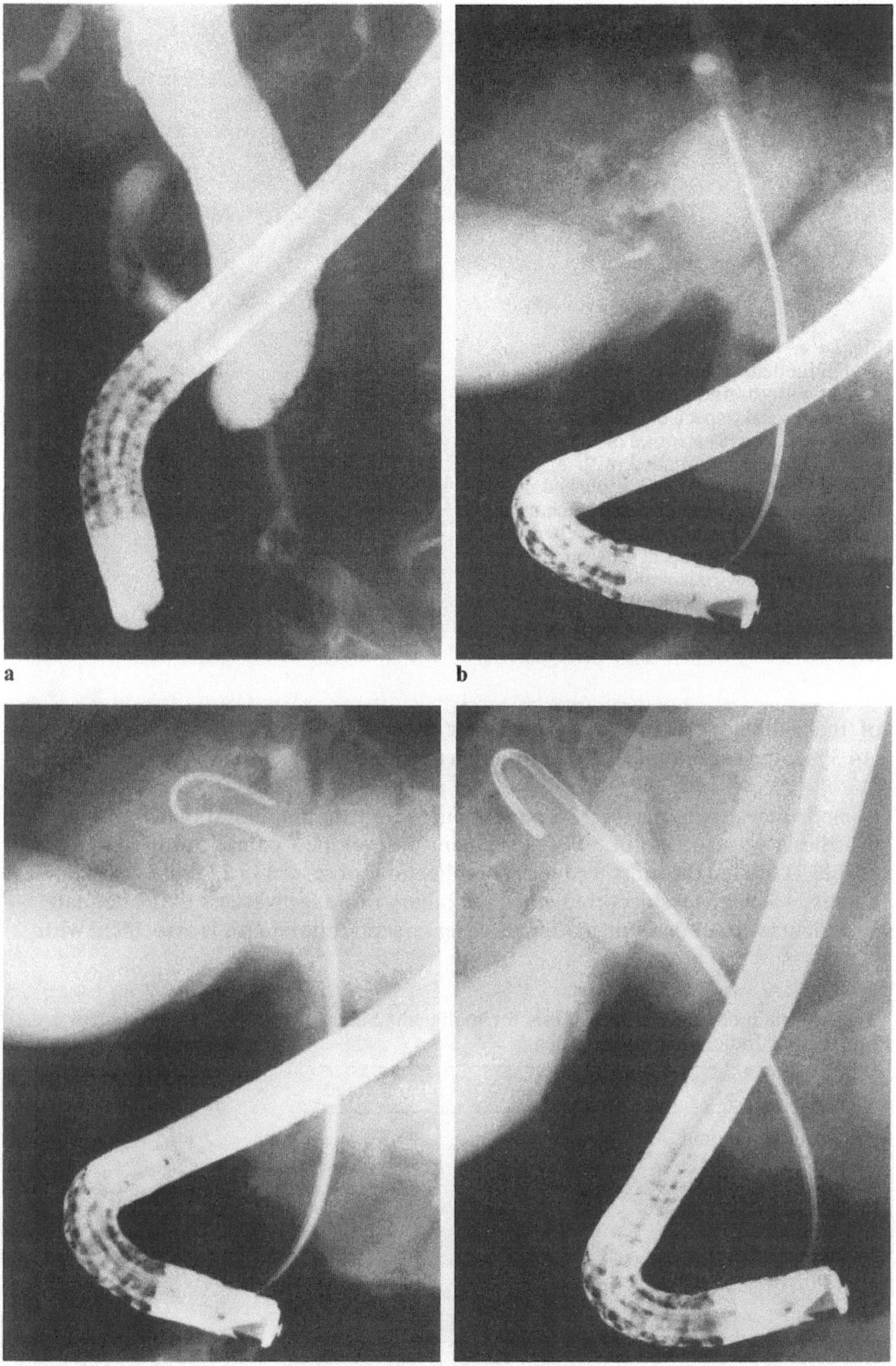

a

b

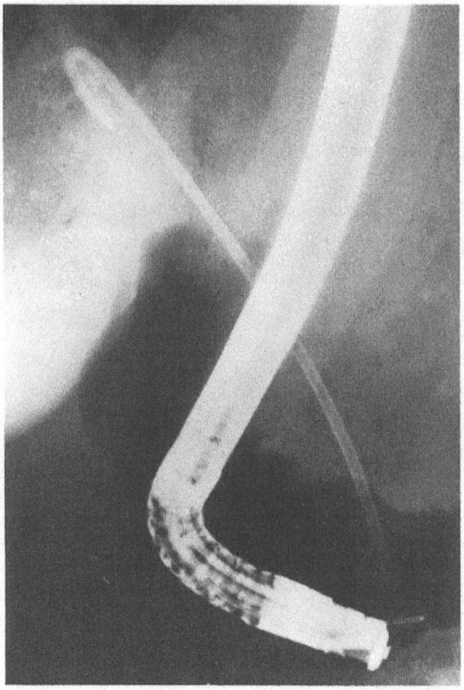

e

**Fig. 2a–e.** Endoscopic implantation of a biliduodenal endoprosthesis in a patient with carcinoma of Vater's papilla. **a** Radiological aspect of the distal common bile duct with stenosis of the papilla. **b** The stenosis is sounded with a guide wire. **c** The endoprosthesis is pushed over the wire through the endoscope channel by means of a pusher tube. **d** When the endoprosthesis has reached its final position, the guide wire is withdrawn. **e** After removing the guide wire and pusher tube, the endoprosthesis remains in place

of the gallbladder (14.9%), primary or metastatic tumors of the liver hilus (14.3%), and carcinoma of Vater's papilla and ampulla (6.7%).

*Complications.* Among the 380 patients in whom the implantation of an endoprosthesis was successful, 100 subsequently developed complications (26.3%) (Table 2). By far the most frequent complication, observed in 77 cases, was cholangitis, which always occurred when the biliary drainage was less than adequate. In patients with underlying malignant disease, septic cholangitis is associated with

**Table 1.** Biliduodenal endoprosthesis for malignant biliary obstruction: Indications in 435 patients

| | *n* | Percentage |
|---|---|---|
| Pancreatic carcinoma | 199 | 45.7 |
| Bile duct carcinoma | 80 | 18.4 |
| Gallbladder carcinoma | 65 | 14.9 |
| Primary or metastatic liver hilus tumor | 62 | 14.3 |
| Carcinoma of papilla or ampulla | 29 | 6.7 |
| Total | 435 | 100 |

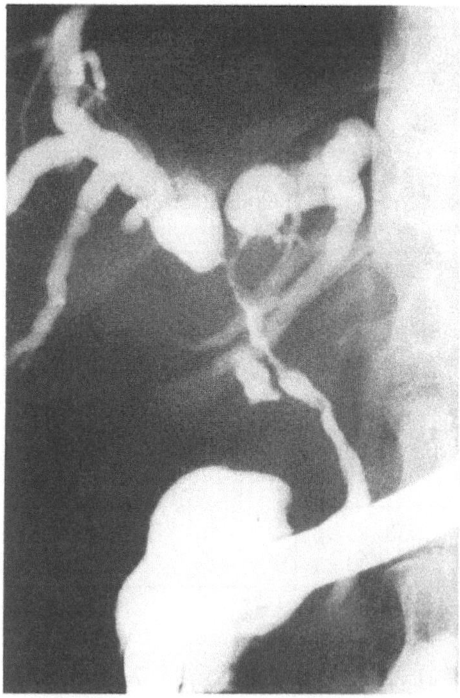

a

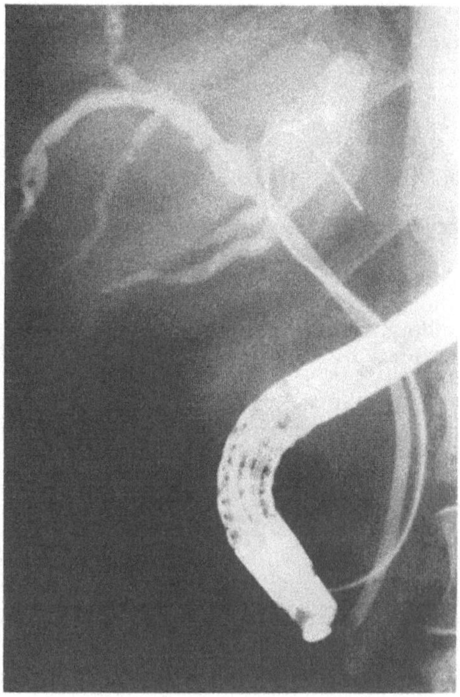

b

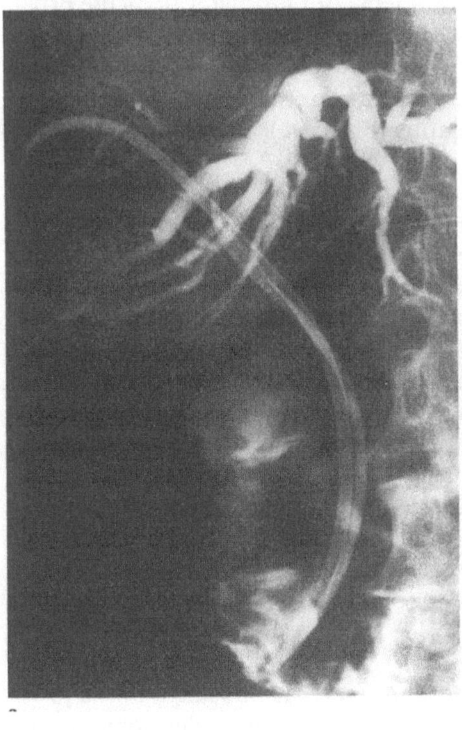

c

**Fig. 4.** Implantation of two biliduodenal endoprostheses in a patient with malignant obstruction of the hepatic bifurcation. **a** Radiological aspect of the biliary duct system. Y-shaped stenosis of the hepatic bifurcation. **b** A biliduodenal endoprosthesis has been implanted in the right liver lobe. Another endoprosthesis is being pushed over the wire into the left hepatic duct. **c** Both of the endoprostheses in situ. Selective drainage of each liver lobe. Contrast medium appearing in the duodenum

**Table 2.** Biliduodenal endoprosthesis for malignant biliary obstruction: Complications in 380 patients

| | Period | | | |
|---|---|---|---|---|
| | 1979 to May 1982 | | Since April 1981 | |
| Complication | *n* | Mortality *n* | Complication rate | Mortality |
| Cholangitis without septicemia | 41 | 2 | | |
| Cholangitis with septicemia | 36 | 20 | | |
| Endoprosthesis dislodgement | 9 | 0 | | |
| Perforation | 6 | 3 | < 10% | < 5% |
| Bleeding | 5 | 2 | | |
| Pancreatitis | 1 | 1 | | |
| Complications unrelated to endoprosthesis | 2 | 2 | | |
| Total | 100 (26.3%) | 30 (7.9%) | | |

a high mortality – 20 of 36 patients (55.6%) died of this condition. More rarely seen complications were dislodgment of the endoprosthesis, bleeding from the papillotomy or the tumor, perforation of the duodenal or bile duct wall by the prosthesis, and acute pancreatitis (Table 2). At 7.9% the mortality was high; this was caused mainly by cholangitis, which was responsible for 73.3% of all the deaths. The next most frequent cause of death was perforation (three cases), followed by hemorrhage (two cases), and acute pancreatitis (one case). Two patients died of causes unrelated to the implantation.

The complication rate of 26.3% and the mortality of 7.9% found in the cases covered by our enquiry are not tolerable. However, these data now have only historical significance and no longer represent the present-day figures. This is due to the fact that they include the complications that developed during the early "pioneering days" of the technique. During this developmental phase, all the working groups had very high complication rates (up to 60%!). In retrospect, these failures may be explained by the use of unsuitable material (small-caliber prostheses), the lack of experience on the part of the endoscopists, and uncertainties vis-á-vis the indication. In the meantime, the complication rates have decreased continually. Following the introduction of the large-caliber endoprosthesis with outside diameters of 10 French, the complication rate in all the working groups dropped to below 10%, and the mortality to below 5% (Table 2). In view of the bad prognosis for malignant diseases of the biliary system and the fact that the majority of the patients concerned are inoperable, this risk would appear to be acceptable.

In the longer course, occlusion of the endoprosthesis by "sludge material," with cell detritus and viscous bile (Fig. 6), regularly occurs. The blockage of the prosthesis leads to a recurrent cholestasis, and cholangitis regularly develops. In this

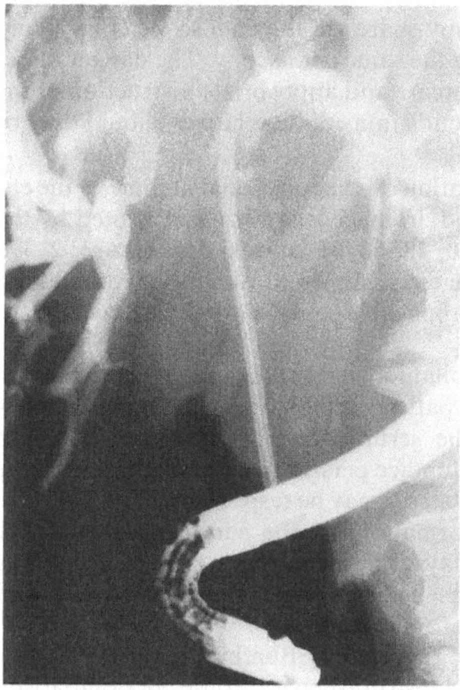

a

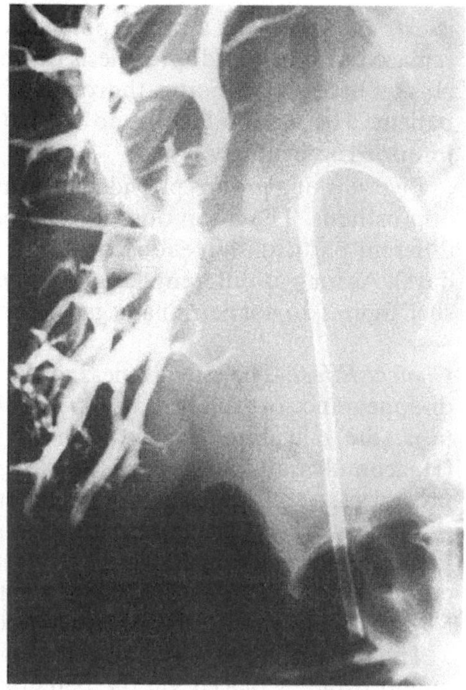

b

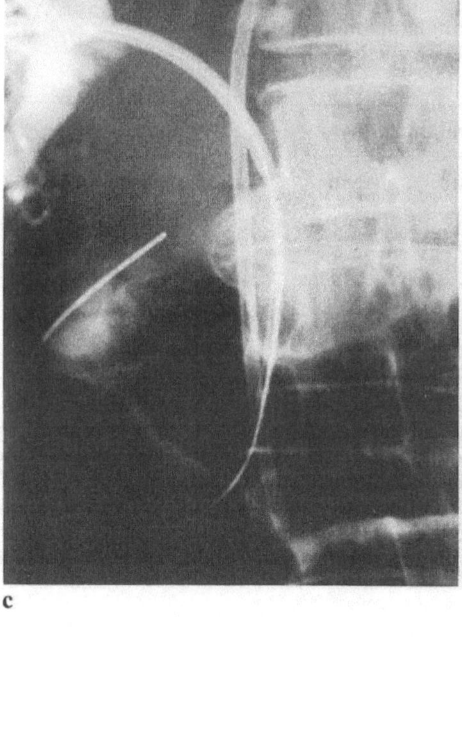

c

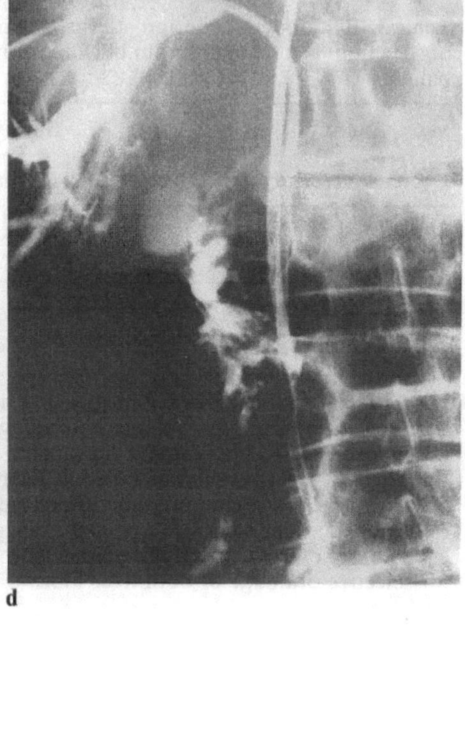

d

situation, immediate removal of the endoprosthesis is indicated. The prosthesis is extracted with the aid of a polypectomy snare via the endoscope (Fig. 7) and replaced by a new endoprosthesis during the same endoscopy. The danger of occlusion necessitates both a thorough aftercare and appropriate instruction of the patient. The family doctor and the patient's immediate relatives should also be informed accordingly.

Five working groups provided information on the functional lifetime of the endoprosthesis. The mean duration of good drainage was variously quoted by the different participating endoscopists as 10, 42, 56, 65, and 96 days (range: 2–390 days). As long as different designs and materials are employed for the prostheses, such figures do not permit any generally applicable conclusions to be drawn.

*Clinical Effect.* The effectiveness of the biliduodenal drainage is indicated by the disappearance of jaundice. In 105 of 121 patients (86.8%) with malignant cholestasis, the bilirubin concentration in the serum dropped by more than half (Hagenmüller and Soehendra 1983). If jaundice persists after implantation of the prosthesis, technical reasons or liver metastases may be responsible.

Three working groups provided information on the survival times of 149 patients. Survival ranged from 1 to 760 days. The mean survival times from three centers were 88, 106, and 112 days, and the median survival times were 47, 74, and 81 days. Only a single patient survivied for 2 years.

The survival times are similar to those reported by Burcharth et al. (1981) for endoprostheses placed via the percutaneous-transhepatic route. In comparison with patients treated surgically by a biliodigestive anastomosis, Burcharth's group of inoperable patients revealed no significantly shorter median survival times. An analysis of 48 patients from our department showed that those in whom serum

**Table 3.** Biliduodenal endoprosthesis for malignant biliary obstruction: Decrease in serum bilirubine and survival of 48 patients

| | | Survival time (days) | |
|---|---|---|---|
| Decrease in serum bilirubine | *n* | Median | Mean |
| <50% | 10 | 21.5 [a] | 24.6 [a] |
| >50% | 38 | 75.5 [a] | 128.8 [a] |

[a] $P<0.05$

◀ **Fig. 5.** Female patient with an obstructing liver hilus metastasis from breast cancer. Combined endoscopic and percutaneous drainage technique. **a** The left liver lobe is drained by an endoscopically implanted biliduodenal endoprosthesis. Endoscopic drainage of the right hepatic duct system has failed. **b** There is no communication between right and left hepatic ducts. Percutaneous puncture of the right hepatic duct system is performed. **c** The right hepatic duct stenosis is passed by a guide wire. An endoprosthesis is pushed percutaneously over the guide wire. **d** Endoscopic and percutaneous endoprosthesis in place for selective drainage of both liver lobes

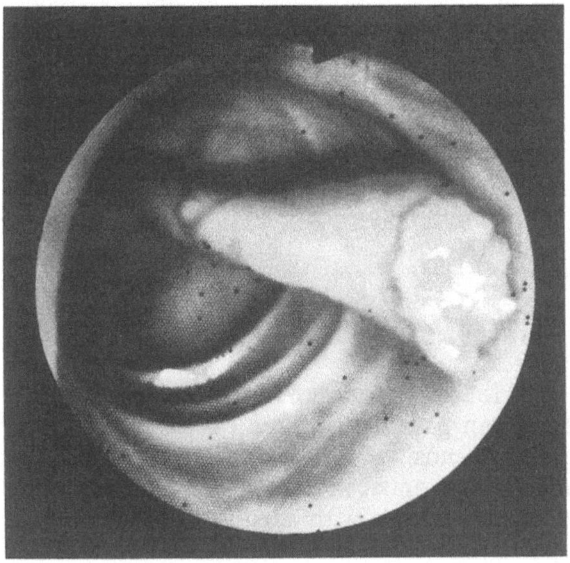

**Fig. 6.** Duodenoscopic aspect of an occluded biliduodenal endoprosthesis

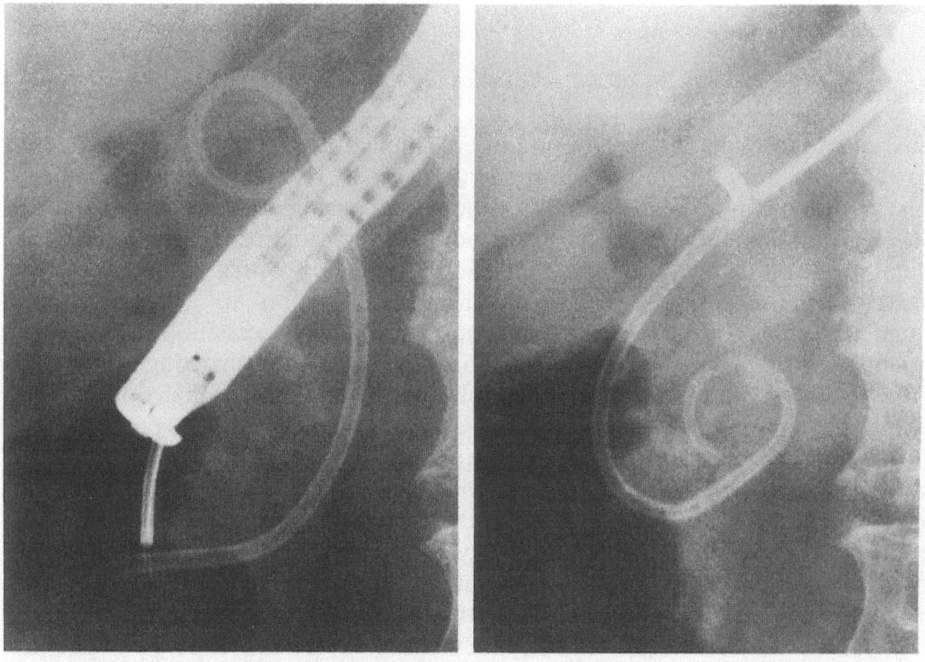

**Fig. 7.** Removal of an occluded biliduodenal endoprosthesis, radiological aspect. Same patient as in Fig. 2. *Left,* The distal tip of the endoprosthesis is grasped with a polypectomy snare; *right,* The endoprosthesis is withdrawn together with the endoscope

**Table 4.** Bilioduodenal endoprosthesis in patients with malignant biliary obstruction: Localisation of the stenosis and survival of 44 patients

| Localisation of the stenosis | Patients *n* | Survival (days) | |
|---|---|---|---|
| | | Mean | Median |
| Ductus hepatocholedochus | 31 | 141.2 | 90 [a] |
| Hepatic bifurcation and/or Ductus hepatici proprii | 13 | 77.1 | 55 [a] |
| Total | 44 | | |

[a] $p<0.01$

bilirubin dropped by more than 50% following endoprosthesis implantation had a significantly longer survival time than patients in whom cholestasis persisted ($P<0.05$, see Table 3). The site of the stenosis within the biliary system did also influence the survival time: Patients with an obstruction of the ductus hepatocholedochus survived longer than patients with stenosis of the hepatic bifurcation and/or the ductus hepatici proprii ($p<0.01$, see Table 4). In contrast, no correlation was found between the survival time and patient age (correlation coefficient $r=-0.12$), serum albumin concentration ($r=0.06$), or serum bilirubin concentration ($r=-0.25$) prior to the implantation. Nor was any statistically significant influence of the presence of metastases on the length of survival observed.

## Summary

Since its introduction in 1979, the endoscopic implantation of biliduodenal endoprostheses has rapidly found widespread acceptance. Its most important indication (in 86% of cases) is obstruction of the biliary passage by malignant tumors. The results of this study show the experience gained by six European specialists in a total of 380 patients in whom implantation of an endoprosthesis was successful. The technical procedure is largely standardized – in contrast to the material and design of the prostheses employed. Implantation is successful in 83.7% of patients. The most frequent indication (45.7% of cases) is obstructing carcinoma of the pancreas, which is in frequency followed by carcinoma of the bile ducts, gallbladder carcinoma, liver hilus tumors, and carcinomas of Vater's papilla.

If the results obtained with the technique during the early days of its application are included, the complication rate is 26.3% (of which cholangitis accounts for 77.3%) and the mortality is 7.9%. In the meantime, the complication rate has dropped to below 10%, and the mortality to below 5%. Occlusion of the endoprosthesis is a problem regularly encountered in aftercare. The endoprosthesis leads to a marked improvement of cholestasis in more than 85% of cases. The average survival times are reported to be between 88 and 142 days; only one patient survived for 2 years. In this respect, the procedure would appear to be equally as effective as percutaneous-transhepatic endoprosthesis implantation and palliative surgery.

## References

Burcharth F, Efsen F, Christiansen LA, Hancke S, Jensen LI, Nielsen OV, Pedersen JH (1981) Nonsurgical internal biliary drainage by endoprosthesis. Surg Gynecol Obstet 153:857–860

Hagenmüller F, Classen M (1982) Therapeutic endoscopic and percutaneous procedures for biliary diseases. In: Popper H, Schaffner F (eds) Progress in liver diseases, vol VII. Grune and Stratton, New York, pp 299–317

Hagenmüller F, Soehendra N (1983) Non-surgical biliary drainage. Saunders, London, pp 297–316 (Clinics in Gastroenterology, vol 12, no 1)

Soehendra N, Reynders-Frederix V (1979) Palliative Gallengangdrainage. Eine neue Methode zur endoskopischen Einführung eines inneren Drains. Dtsch Med Wochenschr 104:206–207

# 17 Balloon Dilatation of Bile Duct Strictures

*J. E. Geenen*

Bakes (1928) reported that ampullary dilatation with a series of dilators, greatly reduced the incidence of residual stones following exploration of the common bile duct. Burhenne (1975) dilated biliary strictures using the sinus tract of a T tube for access to the biliary tree and later the percutaneous transhepatic approach for benign stricture dilatation was added (Burhenne and Morris 1980). Lee et al. (1977) attempted dilatation of a bile duct stricture endoscopically in 1977 through a choledochoduodenostomy, using a Fogarty balloon attached to a forward-viewing panendoscope. Burhenne and Morris (1980) found that stricture dilatation with a Gruntzig balloon catheter (Gruntzig et al. 1973) was more practical and less time-consuming. Vennes and Silvis (1982) and Siegel and Guelrud (1982) reported their initial experiences with dilatation of bile duct, pancreatic duct, and sphincter of Oddi strictures using a side-viewing endoscope and a Gruntzig-type balloon catheter.

Benign biliary tract strictures tend to recur (with a frequency of approximately 30%) after surgical repair, and the availability of a nonoperative approach provides a useful alternative.

Because of the limited reports in the literature (Centola et al. 1981; Martin and Fankuchen 1981; Martin et al. 1980; Molnar and Stockum 1978; Ring et al. 1978; Staritz et al. 1982; Teplick et al. 1980) and the development of a large-channel side-viewing endoscope with suitable Gruntzig balloons, a world-wide survey of physicians performing endoscopic balloon dilatation of pancreatico-biliary duct strictures was undertaken. Ten gastrointestinal endoscopists have reported that they currently dilate strictures using angioplasty-type balloons (Table 1).

## Methods

Balloon dilatation of strictures requires a side-viewing cannulating endoscope with a biopsy channel diameter of 2.8–3.7 mm. The balloon catheters are a modification of angioplasty

**Table 1.** Physicians performing balloon dilatation of stricture

| Names of physicians | Country | Names of physicians | Country |
|---|---|---|---|
| M. Classen, MD | W. Germany | K. Huibregtse, MD | Holland |
| P. Cotton, MD | England | L. Safrany, MD | W. Germany |
| M. Cremer, MD | Belgium | J. Siegel, MD | USA |
| J. Geenen, MD | USA | J. Vennes, MD | USA |
| M. Guelrud, MD | Venezuela | D. Wurbs, MD | W. Germany |

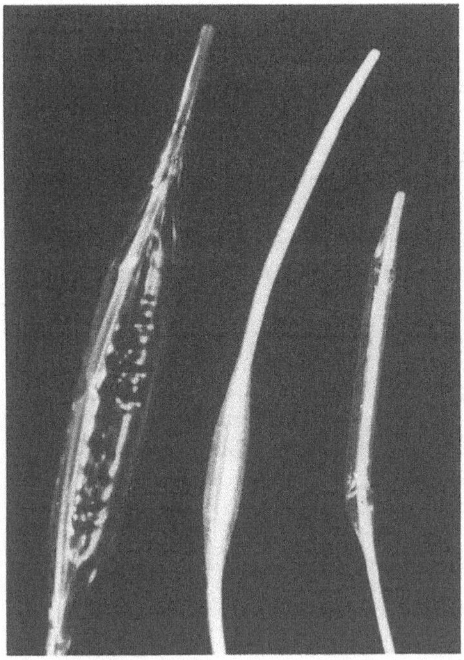

**Fig. 1.** Gruntzig type ballon catheter for dialatation of stricture. (Medi-Techh, Inc., and Cook Inc.)

catheters (Medi-Tech, Inc. and Cook, Inc.) (Fig. 1). These catheters are 5 Fr to 8 Fr in diameter and 180 cm in length. The distended balloon measures 2–4 cm in length, with a diameter of 4–8 mm. Pressure of up to 75 PSI or 5 atm can be generated in the balloon.

Following diagnostic ERCP, a 400-cm coiled-spring guide wire is inserted through the cannula into the appropriate duct proximal to the stricture. Under fluoroscopic control, the cannula is withdrawn over the wire while the position of the guide wire is maintained. Once the cannula is removed the balloon catheter is placed over the guide wire and positioned across the stricture. The balloon is filled with 60% contrast medium under fluoroscopic control. The balloon is fully distended, exerting a pressure of 5 atm for 3 minutes and then deflated. This is repeated twice at each setting. Repeat dilatation is performed if the initial response is inconclusive. In patients with common bile duct stricture, an endoprosthesis can be positioned across the stricture for 1–3 months to promote re-epithelialization of the traumatized duct lumen without restricturing.

## Results

Balloon dilatation of strictures was attempted in 65 patients: there were 27 patients with bile duct strictures, 9 with pancreatic duct strictures, and 29 patients with strictures of the sphincter of Oddi (Table 2). The types of balloons most frequently used were manufactured by Medi-Tech, Inc. or Cook Inc. Two physicians used the Edwards balloon, and one physician constructed his own balloon. The size of the catheter was either 5 Fr or 7 Fr and the diameter of the balloon varied from 4 mm to 15 mm (self-made).

Balloon dilatation was successful in 18 of 27 patients with bile duct stricture (Table 3). Postoperative bile duct strictures were the most common type, followed by malignant bile duct strictures.

Pancreatic duct strictures were limited to strictures of the main pancreatic duct in the head (Table 4). One patient with pancreatitis thought to be secondary to pancreatic divisum had successful dilatation of the pancreatic duct through the minor papilla.

Balloon dilatation of strictures of the sphincter of Oddi segment was successful in 29 of 30 patients (Table 5). In several patients restenosed sphincter segments after endoscopic sphincterotomy were successfully dilated.

In this survey there were six complications following balloon dilatation (9.2%). Five patients developed mild pancreatitis and one patient developed cholangitis (Table 6).

**Table 2.** Sites of stricture relieved by balloon dilatation ($n=65$)

| Site | Bile duct | Pancreatic duct | Sphincter of Oddi |
|---|---|---|---|
| No. of Patients | 27 | 9 | 29 |

**Table 3.** Attempted balloon dilatation of biliary tree stricture

| Type of stricture | Attempts | Successful |
|---|---|---|
| Inflammatory (idiopathic) | 4 | 2 |
| Postoperative | 10 | 9 |
| Sclerosing cholangitis | 4 | 2 |
| Choledochoduodenostomy | 2 | 2 |
| Malignant | 7 | 3 |
| Totals | 27 | 18 |

**Table 4.** Attempted balloon dilatation of pancreatic duct (PD) strictures

| Types | Attempts | Successful |
|---|---|---|
| Main PD | 7 | 5 |
| Pancreatic divisum | 1 | 1 |
| Totals | 8 | 6 |

**Table 5.** Attempted balloon dilatation of stricture of sphincter of Oddi segment (SO)

| Types | Attemts | Succesful |
|---|---|---|
| SO dysfunction | 25 | 24 |
| Stricture at CBD orifice (post ES) | 4 | 4 |
| Stricture at PD orifice (post ES) | 1 | 1 |
| Totals | 30 | 29 |

**Table 6.** Complications of balloon dilatation of stricture (65 patients)

| Complication | Number |
|---|---|
| Sepsis | 1 |
| Bleeding | 0 |
| Perforation | 0 |
| Pancreatitis | 5 |
| Total | 6 |

In conclusion, the results achieved which endoscopic Gruntzig balloon dilatation of pancreatico-biliary duct strictures appear encouraging, and this procedure is associated with a low complication rate. However, this survey is exclusively retrospective, and there was only a short follow-up period in most patients. The long-term results of balloon dilatation of benign bile duct strictures in a few patients substantiate the potential value of this procedure for a select group of patients. Prospective multicenter clinical trials, with several years' follow-up, are desirable before balloon dilatation of strictures becomes a routine clinical procedure.

## References

Bakes J (1928) On the drainage-less surgery of the bile passages and on the methodical dilatation of the papilla. Zentralbl Chir 55:1858
Burhenne HJ (1975) Dilatation of biliary tract strictures. A new roentgenologic technique. Radiol Clin North Am 44:153–159
Burhenne HJ, Morris DC (1980) Biliary stricture dilatation: use of the Gruntzig balloon catheter. J Can Assoc Radiol 31:196–197
Centola CAP, Jander HJ et al. (1981) Balloon dilatation of papilla of Vater to allow biliary stone passage. Am J Radiol 136:613–614
Gruntzig A, Bollinger A et al. (1973) Perkutane Rekanalisation chronischer arterieller Verschlüsse nach Dotter – eine nicht operative Kathetertechnik. Schweiz Med Wochenschr 103:825–831
Lee TG, Katon R et al. (1977) Endoscopic retrograde cholangiodilatation: a preliminary report. Gastrointest Endosc 23:171–172
Martin EC, Fankuchen EI (1981) Percutaneous dilatation in primary sclerosing cholangitis: two experiences. Am J Radiol 137:603–605
Martin EC, Karlson KB et al. (1980) Percutaneous transhepatic dilatation of intrahepatic biliary stricutes. Am J Radiol 135:837–840
Molnar W, Stockum AE (1978) Transhepatic dilatation of choledochoenterostomy strictures. Radiology 129:59–64
Ring EJ, Oleaga JA et al. (1978) Therapeutic application of catheter cholangiography. Radiology 128:333–338
Siegel JH, Guelrud M (1982) Endoscopic cholangioplasty: Hydrostatic dilatation in pancreatico-biliary diseases. Gastrointest Endosc 28:144 (Abstract)
Staritz M, Ewe K et al. (1982) Endoscopic papillary dilatation, a possible alternative to endoscopic papillotomy. Lancet I:1306–1307
Teplick SK, Goldstein RC et al. (1980) Percutaneous transhepatic choledochoplasty and dilatation of cholechoenterostomy strictures. JAMA 244:1240–1242
Vennes JA, Silvis SE (1982) Endoscopic retrograde balloon dilatation. Gastrointest Endosc 28:149 (Abstract)

# 18 Endoscopic Bile Drainage: Discussion, Summary

*P. B. Cotton*

The panel first addressed the problem of large stones, highlighted by Leuschner's presentation on chemical dissolution. Results had been particularly disappointing with primary stones. Hofmann reported that new agents were being developed, but emphasized their potential toxicity. More encouraging results were reported with the use of a mechanical lithotriptor, snare loops, and the Nd-Yag laser (in Japan). Many groups were using endoprostheses in patients with irremovable stones, but detailed results were not available.

The panel then discussed endoscopic balloon dilatation in the bile duct, as presented by Geenen. Several groups had shown objective effects on sphincter activity (by manometry and radiology), but it was too early to assess clinical results. Balloon dilatation of strictures remained experimental.

The panel fully endorsed the routine use of endoscopic sphincterotomy for the removal of common duct stones, which is now widely practiced throughout the world. Few groups find it necessary to employ endoscopic diathermy choledochoduodenostomy, as advocated by Machado. All groups used nasobiliary drainage in patients with acute cholangitis, and as interval management between attempts at removing large stones.

Nasobiliary drainage was rarely used in patients with malignant obstruction, but there was rapidly increasing interest and experience with endoscopic endoprostheses. The reviews by Huibregtse and Hagenmüller showed high success rates, but a substantial problem with tube blockage and cholangitis – particularly in patients with hilar lesions. Many different sizes, shapes and designs of prosthesis are being used. Panel discussion did not identify any consensus about optimal design, or whether long-term antibiotics or choloretics were effective in preventing late obstruction. Limited experience with endoscopic endoprosthesis in patients with benign stenosis (strictures and sclerosing cholangitis) warranted further experimentation.

There was full agreement that the endoscopic transpapillary approach to biliary obstruction is effective in many areas, and has major development potential. However, the panel identified many problems for further study:

1. How often is it possible to determine that a tumor is nonresectable without surgery?
2. What proportion of patients with pancreatic tumors develop duodenal obstruction after biliary bypass?
3. Are there particular patients who are more suitable for surgical bypass or a percutaneous approach?

4. What are the optimum characteristics for a prosthesis, and how are they best maintained? Should they be changed routinely?

The Chairman concluded by recommending prospective studies of these problems to provide answers as quickly as possible and reminded the panel and audience that, in patients with malignant jaundice, the aim was to provide relatively short-term palliation; the patients' interests were not necessarily best served by technical gymnastics, particularly if they had to be repeated frequently.

# IV. Disturbances After Biliary Drainage

# 19 Infective Complications

*E. B. Helm and W. Stille*

## Introduction

The different techniques of biliary drainage may be lifesaving by releasing biliary obstruction in certain patients – mainly those with biliary tumor (Wurbs and Classen 1977). Nevertheless, new techniques may lead to new types of complications (Bilbao et al. 1976; Davis et al. 1974; Koch 1979; Mason 1968; Silvis et al. 1976). The different methods for nonsurgical biliary drainage carry a marked risk of bacterial complications, mainly the development of septicemia (Helm et al. 1983).

In our hospital we evaluated the risk of bacterial infection by series of cultures in patients undergoing ERC (endoscopic retrograde cholangiography) with or without biliary drainage. In all patients with temperature ≧38 °C, blood cultures were done as a routine procedure. Due to the large numbers of ERCs performed and the numerous patients with biliary obstruction, we are able to report on several septicemia cases as a typical complication of ERC and biliary drainage.

## Method

Biliary samples were collected before administration of x-ray medium in the course of ERC. The samples were inoculated within 2 hours on adequate media (EMB, blood agar etc.). Two blood culture bottles (Biotest) were cultured under aerobic and anaerobic conditions in the event of fever (≧38 °C).

## Results

Biliary infections have a typical spectrum of pathogens (Table 1). Microbiological studies of bile samples collected during surgical procedures demonstrated an almost identical spectrum of bacteria. *E. coli* was the predominant pathogen, followed by various *Streptococci* species. *Pseudomonas aeruginosa* did not play a major role as pathogen in biliary infections in the pre-ERC era (Bergan et al. 1979; England and Rosenblatt 1977; Keighly et al. 1974, 1975; Knothe et al. 1977; Mason 1968; Wacha and Helm 1982).

Our own results relating to biliary septicemia correlated well with these findings; *Pseudomonas aeruginosa* was isolated in only two cases (Table 2) (Shah et al. 1976).

When analysing the spectrum of pathogens in bile collected from patients undergoing ERC, we noted differences with regard to common findings in biliary infections. ERC patients had a high percentage of *Pseudomonas aeruginosa;*

**Table 1.** Pathogens isolated from intraoperative bile (Helm et al., 1982)

| | Mason 1968 | Keighly 1974, 1975 | Knothe 1976 | England 1977 | Wacha 1979 | Bergan 1979 |
|---|---|---|---|---|---|---|
| *E. coli* | 25 | 29 | 18 | 169 | 25 | 16 |
| *Klebsiella* sp. | 7 | 8 | 2 | 116 | 10 | 8 |
| *Enterobacter* sp. | | 2 | | 32 | 8 | |
| *Pseudomonas* sp. | 2 | 1 | 2 | 65 | 2 | |
| Other Gram-negative bacilli | 7 | | 2 | 20 | 12 | 1 |
| *Proteus* sp. | | | | 43 | | |
| *Staph. epidermidis* | | 1 | 9 | 22 | 5 | |
| *Staph. aureus* | 9 | 1 | 2 | 7 | 3 | |
| *Streptococcus faecalis* | | | 13 | 132 | 14 | 4 |
| Other *Streptococcus* sp. | 5 | 7 | 27 | 46 | 17 | 4 |
| Other Gram-positive bacilli | | | | 48 | | |
| *Clostridia* sp. | 7 | | 2 | 61 | | |
| Bacteroides | | | | 78 | 2 | |

**Table 2.** Spectrum of bacteria isolated from blood cultures from 44 patients with biliary septicemia before availability of ERC (Helm et al., 1982)

| Pathogens | *N* |
|---|---|
| *E. coli* | 22 |
| *E. coli* + *Streptococcus faecalis* | 1 |
| *Streptococcus* sp. | 6 |
| *Streptococcus faecalis* | 3 |
| *Klebsiella/Enterobacter* | 3 |
| *Salmonella* sp. | 3 |
| *Ps. aeruginosa* | 2 |
| *Proteus mirabilis* | 2 |
| *Staphylococcus aureus* | 1 |
| *Corynebacterium* sp. | 1 |
| *Bacteroides fragilis* | 1 |

mixed infections were frequent (Table 3). Gram-positive and anaerobic bacteria were rare and are not mentioned in Table 3.

The spectrum of pathogens in septicemia following ERC was different from the spectrum in patients with biliary infections who had not undergone endoscopic procedures (Table 4). Following ERC, *Pseudomonas aeruginosa* was more frequent than *E. coli*.

The great majority of the patients with septicemia in the course of biliary drainage (27 of 32) suffered from biliary tumor. There was a distinct correlation between *Pseudomonas* septicemia and tumor (Table 5).

Many patients were admitted to our hospital for endoscopic biliary drainage because the severity of their condition did not allow surgical decompression. The prevalence of *Pseudomonas aeruginosa* in biliary septicemia is even more pro-

**Table 3.** Bacteriological results in bile samples taken from 142 patients during ERCP (Helm at al., 1982)

| | *E. coli* | *Klebs./ entero-bacter* | *Pseudo-monas aeruginosa* | Others | Sterile | Total number of patients with mono- or mixed cultures |
|---|---|---|---|---|---|---|
| Monocultures | 36 | 4 | 24 | 2 | | 66 (46%) |
| Mixed cultures (2 different bacteria) | 45 | 27 | 26 | 4 | | 51 (36%) |
| Mixed cultures (3 different bacteria) | 8 | | 8 | 8 | | 8 (5.6%) |
| Sterile | | | | | 17 | 17 (12%) |
| Total | 89 | 31 | 58 | 14 | 17 | 142 (100%) |
| Cultures which contained above-mentioned bacteria | 62.7% | 21.8% | 40.8% | 2.8% | 12% 12% | |

**Table 4.** Spectrum of pathogens of septicemia in the course of ERCP (Frankfurt, ZIM 1.4.1979 to 31.5.1982) (Helm et al., 1982)

| | Polymicrobial infection | Monoinfection | Total |
|---|---|---|---|
| *PS. aeruginosa* | 6 | 12 | 18 |
| *E. coli* | 4 | 9 | 13 |
| *Str. faecalis* | 4 | 3 | 7 |
| *Citrobacter* | 2 | 1 | 3 |
| *Klebsiella* | 1 | 5 | 6 |
| *Serratia* | – | 1 | 1 |
| *Proteus* sp. | 1 | 1 | 2 |
| *Bacteroides* sp. | 1 | – | 1 |
| "Nonfermenters" | – | 2 | 2 |
| Total | 19 | 34 | 53 |

nounced if the bacterial spectrum in patients with polymicrobial septicemia is included in this analysis.

Of 9 patients with polymicrobial septicemia, 7 had malignant obstructions. In 6 patients suffering from tumor, *Pseudomonas aeruginosa* was one of the pathogens isolated in blood cultures (Table 6). In 15 of 32 patients with septicemia and biliary drainage, *Pseudomonas aeruginosa* was present. In total, this pathogen was cultured in 17 of 18 patients with biliary malignancies after ERC.

Septicemia in the course of biliary drainage usually occurred within the first few days after the endoscopic procedure (Table 7). In patients with bilioduodenal

**Table 5.** Spectrum of pathogens of septicemia in the course of ERCP (Frankfurt, ZIM 1.4.1979 to 31.5.1982) (Helm et al. 1982)

| | Biliary drainage | | No drainage | | |
|---|---|---|---|---|---|
| Pathogens | Tumor | Non-tumor | Tumor | Non-tumor | Total |
| *E. coli* | 6 | 1 | – | 2 | 9 |
| *Klebsiella/Enterobacter* | 1 | 3 | 1 | – | 5 |
| *Citrobacter* | 1 | – | – | – | 1 |
| *Serratia marcescens* | 1 | – | – | – | 1 |
| *Proteus mirabilis* | – | – | 1 | – | 1 |
| "Nonfermenter" | 1 | 1 | – | – | 2 |
| *Ps. aeruginosa* | 11 | – | – | 1 | 12 |
| *Str. faecalis* | 1 | – | – | 2 | 3 |
| Polymicrobial | 5 | – | 2 | 2 | 9 |
| Total | 27 | 5 | 4 | 7 | 43 |

**Table 6.** Polymicrobial septicemia in the course of ERCP (Helm et al. 1982)

| | Patient | Tumor | Pathogen | Death |
|---|---|---|---|---|
| No drainage | 1. R. 84 years | – | *E. coli* + *Bacteroides* sp. | 0 |
| | 2. E. 69 years | – | *E. coli* + *Str. faecalis* | + |
| | 3. L. 84 years | + | *Ps. aeruginose* + *Klebsiella* | + |
| | 4. B. 68 years | + | *Ps. aeruginosa* *Str. faecalis* | + |
| Nasobiliary drainage | 5. S. 76 years | + | *Citrobacter* + *Str. faecalis* | 0 |
| Endoprothesis | 6. M. 48 years | + | *Ps. aeruginosa* + *Str. faecalis* | 0 |
| | 7. M. 48 years | + | *Ps. aeruginosa* | 0 |
| | | | *E. coli* + *Proteus mirabilis* | + |
| | 8. R. 66 years | + | *Ps. aeruginosa* + *E. coli* | + |
| | 9. H. 78 years | + | *Ps. aeruginosa* + *Citrobacter* | |

endoprothesis, occlusion of the tube some weeks after insertion was quite common.

The mortality of patients with biliary drainage and septicemia is relatively high. Nine of 32 patients with septicemia died in the acute phase (Table 8). There was no strict correlation between mortality and bacterial species, but there was a correlation between the type of obstruction and the outcome. None of the patients with benign obstruction died of septicemia.

**Table 7.** Emergence of septicemia after ERCP with nasobiliary drainage or bilioduodenal endoprothesis or percutaneous biliary drainage (Helm et al. 1982)

| Days after endoscopic procedure | 0 | 1 | 2 | 3 | 4 | 5 | 6 | 7 | Late | *N* |
|---|---|---|---|---|---|---|---|---|---|---|
| Nasobiliary | 2 | 5 | 3 | 2 | 2 | 1 | – | 1 | – | 16 |
| Endoprothesis | 1 | 1 | 1 | 1 | 1 | – | – | – | 6 | 11 |
| Percutaneous | 1 | – | 1 | 1 | – | – | 1 | – | 1 | 5 |
| Total | 4 | 6 | 5 | 4 | 3 | 1 | 1 | 1 | 7 | 32 |

**Table 8.** Mortality connected with septicemia among 32 patients with biliary drainage (Helm et al. 1982)

| Pathogen | Total | Death |
|---|---|---|
| *E. coli* | 7 | 2 |
| *Klebsiella/ Enterobacter* | 4 | – |
| *Citrobacter* | 1 | – |
| *Serratia* | 1 | 1 |
| Nonfermenter | 2 | 1 |
| *Ps. aeruginosa* | 11 | 3 |
| *Str. faecalis* | 1 | – |
| Polymicrobial | 5 | 2 |
| Total | 32 | 9 |

## Conclusions

Septicemia in connection with biliary drainage is a new complication of modern medical techniques, but no precise reports on this kind of complications are as yet available in the literature.

Our data on the spectrum of bacteria in patients with biliary drainage demonstrate the change in the predominant pathogen from *E. coli* to *Pseudomonas aeruginosa* in septicemia following ERC. It is too easy to explain the prevalence of *Pseudomonas* as ordinary cross-infection. Undoubtedly, the quality of sterilization of endoscopes plays a part in the pathogenesis, but tumor, obstruction, and foreign bodies should not be neglected. In our opinion, small quantities of *Ps. aeruginosa* can easily be introduced into the biliary tract by the endoscopic procedure. In patients with obstruction and biliary tumor *Pseudomonas* can easily become a permanent inhabitant of the biliary tract, with septicemia developing as a consequence. There are several other examples of the coincidence of local necrosis, local tumor, and also foreign bodies causing *Pseudomonas* infection (Strand et al. 1982).

On the other hand, septicemia attributable to *Pseudomonas aeruginosa* following ERC is a new disease. Besides burns, leukemia, intravenous devices, and chronic urological infections, ERC and biliary drainage play an important part as the portal of entry of septicemia due to *Pseudomonas*. In our hospital this was the most frequent pathogenesis of *Pseudomonas* septicemia in the last year.

The high risk of septicemia in biliary drainage makes intensive antibacterial chemotherapy and probably also antibiotic prophylaxis mandatory. The usual antibiotics given for biliary infections are not effective against *Pseudomonas aeruginosa*. Non specific emergency treatment or prophylaxis should be performed with agents which attain high levels in the bile even in case of obstruction and have a broad spectrum of activity, being active against *Pseudomonas*.

Piperacillin, mezlocillin, cefotaxim, cefoperazon, and moxalactam fulfil these requirements. The chemotherapy administered in the presence of biliary drainage should be adapted to the specific spectrum of pathogens, which differs markedly from conventional biliary infections. Controlled studies on the effect of antibiotics under these conditions are urgently necessary.

## References


Bergan T, Dobloug I, Liavag I (1979) Bacterial isolates in cholecystitis and cholelithiasis. Scand J Gastroenterol 14:625–631

Bilbao MK, Dotter CT, Lee TG, Katon RM (1976) Complications of endoscopic retrogade cholangiopancreatography. Gastroenterology 70:314–320

Davis J, Milligan F, Cameran J (1974) Septic complications following endoscopic retrograde cholangiopancreatography. Surg Gynecol Obstet 140:365

England DM, Rosenblatt JE (1977) Anaerobes in human biliary tracts. J Clin Microbiol 6:494–496

Greene WH, Mody M, Harley M, Effman R, Aisner E, Young J, Wiernick RH (1974) Esophagoscopy as a source of *Pseudomonas aeruginosa* sepsis in patients with acute leukemia: the need for sterilization of endoscopes. Gastroenterology 5:912

Helm EB, Hagenmüller F, Stille W (1983) Septikämie nach Eingriffen am Gallengangssystem. MMW 125:210–212

Keighly MRB, Lister DM, Jacobs SI, Giles GR (1974) Hazards of surgical treatment due to microorganisms in the bile. Surgery 75:578–583

Keighly MRB, Drysdale RB, Quoraishi H, Burdon DW, Alexander-Williams J (1975) Antibiotic treatment of biliary sepsis. Surg Clin North 55:1379–1390

Knothe H, Maroske D, Wache H (1977) Bakteriologie von Gallenwegsinfektionen. In: Stille W, Timmler R (eds) Verhandlungen der Internationalen Arbeitstagung Gallenwegs-Infektionen. Steinkopf, Darmstadt, pp 54–59

Koch H (1979) Komplikationen der ERCP und deren Verhütung. Endoskopisch retrograde Cholangio-Pankreatikographie – ERCP. L. Demling, H. Koch, W. Rösch, Schattauer, Stuttgart

Mason GR (1968) Bacteriology and antibiotic selection in biliary surgery. Arch Surg 97:533–537

Nebel OT, Silvis SE, Rogers G, Sugawa C, Mandelstam P (1975) Complications associated with endoscopic retrograde cholangiopancreatography. Gastrointestinal Endoscopy 22:14–16

O'Connor BH, Bennett JR, Alexander JG, Sutton DR, Leighton J (1982) Salmonellosis infection transmitted by fibreoptic endoscopes. Lancet II:864

Shah PM, Helm EB, Stille W (1977) Die cholangitische Sepsis. In: Stille W, Timmler R (eds) Verhandlungen der Internationalen Arbeitstagung Gallenweg Infektionen. Steinkopf, Darmstadt, pp 68–69

Silvis ES, Nebel OT, Rogers G, Sugawa C, Mandelstam P (1976) Endoscopic complications: Results of the 1974 American Society for Gastrointestinal Endoscopy survey. JAMA 235:928–930
Strand CL, Bryant JK, Morgan JW, Forster JG, McDonald HP, Morgenstein StL (1982) Nosocomial *Pseudomonas aeruginosa* urinary tract infections. JAMA 248:1815
Wacha H, Helm EB (1982) Efficacy of antibiotics in bacteriobilia. J Antimicrob Chemother 9 [Suppl A]:131–137
Wurbs H, Classen M (1977) Transpapillary long-standing tube for hepatobiliary drainage. Endoscopy 9:192–193

# 20 The Bile-Loss Syndrome: A Doubtful Entity

*A. F. Hofmann*

## Introduction

The term "bile loss syndrome" may be applied to a syndrome of suboptimal health, occurring in patients with a biliary fistula. In this brief editorial the biochemical and physiological consequences of a permanent biliary fistula will be discussed. The approach will be theoretical and analytical, rather than experiential, because the author has not cared for such patients and is rather skeptical that such a syndrome exists.

## The Setting

A permanent biliary fistula is only established in a patient in whom the flow of bile is obstructed. In the majority of instances the obstruction is neoplastic, and treatment may have involved chemotherapy or radiotherapy or both. Therefore, the typical patient with a chronic biliary fistula has underlying and often progressive disease; disease progression may complicate evaluation of the patient and cause the physician to attribute the patient's poor health status to bile loss when it is in fact a direct consequence of the patient's underlying disease.

## Functions of Bile

Bile is a concentrated micellar solution which serves as a vehicle for the excretion of cholesterol and bilirubin, certain heavy metals, and amphipathic drug metabolites (Hofmann 1965; Carey 1979). Bile also has functional properties. The bile acids accelerate the absorption of triglyceride digestion products and are essential for the absorption of fat-soluble vitamins (Thompson and Dietschy 1981). The bicarbonate in bile may play a modest role in maintaining the alkalinity of jejunal content. Bile acids may also have a bacteriostatic effect in the small intestine (Binder et al. 1975), and probably are a major endogenous cathartic (Hofmann 1977 a).

Bile also serves as a transport vehicle for conjugates of vitamin D (Kumar et al. 1980), and an enterohepatic circulation of both folic acid (Steinberg et al. 1979) and vitamin $B_{12}$ (Green et al. 1981) is believed to occur. It should also be noted that certain drugs, such as phenolphthalein laxatives, are absorbed from the small intestine, pass to the liver where they are conjugated with glucuronic acid, are excreted in bile and then not reabsorbed from the small intestine (Colburn 1979). Thus, bile serves as a transport vehicle for drugs which are conjugated in the liver and then excreted into the small intestine, but do not have a true enterohepatic circulation.

Other substances which occur in bile in relatively high concentrations are glutathione, lecithin, and calcium.

## Possible Consequences of a Biliary Fistula

### *1 Loss of Excretory Components of Bile*

The lipids, cholesterol, and bilirubin will be lost in a manner which differs only quantitatively from that in health. When the enterohepatic circulation is intact, about one-fourth of biliary cholesterol is reabsorbed and three-fourths is lost (Borgstrom 1969; Tangedahl et al. 1979). With a biliary fistula there should be no cholesterol absorption, but there should be complete elimination of biliary cholesterol and no absorption of dietary cholesterol. This should have no metabolic significance, however. The loss of bilirubin should also have no metabolic significance. The situation with respect to trace metals such as copper is more complex. In health, excretion via bile maintains total body balance, since copper and probably other trace metals which are excreted in bile are not reabsorbed during intestinal transit (Owen 1964). If, however, bile acids play a role in accelerating the absorption of trace metals, the existence of a biliary fistula will mean that subnormal absorption occurs. If there is an obligate biliary loss, then in principle a trace metal deficiency could occur.

### *2 Loss of Functional or Possibly Functional Components of Bile*

The bile acids are the major constituents of bile. As noted, they play a key role in lipid digestion and absorption, and may also play a role in catharsis. Accordingly, the major consequence of a biliary fistula is a bile acid deficiency in the small and large intestines. The deficiency is much greater in the small intestine, because the enterohepatic circulation is responsible for an extremely large bile acid secretion with each meal.

In the absence of bile acids in the small intestine, the products of fat digestion, fatty acids, and monoglyceride cannot be solubilized in micellar form. As a consequence, they only achieve their true molecular solubility, which is extremely low. The rate of their absorption is greatly slowed, as diffusion through the unstirred layer becomes rate-limiting. Fatty acid absorption spreads throughout the entire small intestine, and unabsorbed fatty acids pass into the large intestine (Knoebel 1972). Fat-soluble vitamins are considered to have virtually no absorption in the absence of bile acids. In a dog with a chronic biliary fistula the first detectable vitamin deficiency is that of vitamin K, which is manifested by severe hypoprothrombinemia (Whipple and Hawkins 1935). A syndrome of vitamin E deficiency associated with neurological abnormality has been identified in children with prolonged biliary obstruction (Rosenblum et al. 1981). Presumably vitamin A is also malabsorbed.

It seems unlikely that the loss of lecithin in a biliary fistula would be of importance. With interruption of the enterohepatic circulation, not more than 3 mmol/

day of lecithin should be lost, and this should easily be replaced by dietary lecithin. It is possible that in the absence of any dietary choline intake a choline deficiency could occur.

Both vitamin $B_{12}$ and folic acid are considered to have enterhepatic circulations. To the best of my knowledge, neither a vitamin $B_{12}$ nor a folic acid deficiency has been reported in patients with chronic biliary fistula, but the possibility of such a deficiency occurring should be entertained, and red blood cell morphology should be examined at regular intervals. Body storages of vitamin $B_{12}$ are usually great, but if the patient has a prolonged biliary fistula, it may be necessary to determine a serum vitamin $B_{12}$ level. Indeed, Whipple attempted to correct the megaloblastic anemia occurring in his biliary fistula dogs by feeding whole liver, and these historic experiments led to the discovery of a treatment for pernicious anemia, the identification of vitamin $B_{12}$, and a Nobel Prize (Whipple 1965).

Other biliary constituents, such as glutathione, will be lost; but this should have little effect on overall glutathione metabolism in the body.

### Fluid and Electrolyte Loss

Fluid and electrolyte loss can be considerable from a biliary fistula. The major anions lost, other than bile acids, will be chloride and bicarbonate. Obviously a metabolic acidosis can occur.

The literature suggests that there are rare patients who experience extraordinary, continuing, and even life-threatening, choleresis following relief of biliary obstruction (Dumont 1982). It is not clear whether the origin of this secretion is at the level of the canaliculus or of the biliary ductules. However, it is clear that it is an electrolyte fraction, and is not bile salt dependent (Bode et al. 1979).

### Altered Drug Metabolism

As noted, certain drugs, such as the cathartic agent phenolphthalein, are absorbed passively in the small intestine, pass to the liver where they are conjugated with glucuronic acid, and are excreted into bile (Colburn 1979). In the presence of the biliary fistula, such compounds will be absorbed and excreted in bile and not enter the small intestine. Therefore, they will be devoid of cathartic activity. Other drugs having an important enterohepatic circulation are certain of the digitalis derivatives. The presence of a biliary fistula should greatly increase the "metabolic disposition" of such compounds. Again, the digitalis requirement might increase considerably in a patient with an external biliary fistula.

### Altered Hormone Metabolism

The sex steroids are excreted in bile in the form of their sulfate and glucuronide conjugates (Adlercreutz et al. 1979). The estrogen conjugates are reabsorbed, so that a biliary fistula could have an important influence on estrogen metabolism. Experiments are needed.

### Induced Changes in Hepatic Metabolism

There is no evidence to suggest that the enterohepatic circulation of bile acids is beneficial to the liver. Bile salts do "down-regulate" cholesterol and bile acid synthesis, so that in the absence of enterohepatic return, cholesterol and bile acid synthesis should increase to the maximum (Dowling et al. 1970; Hofmann 1977b). The magnitude of this increase is 5- to 10-fold and it should have no metabolic significance. Patients with severe ileal dysfunction may have this magnitude of cholesterol and bile acid synthesis for years without apparent consequence. The dog with a chronic biliary fistula is quite healthy, provided vitamin supplementation is given (Pertsemlidis et al. 1973).

It seems unlikely that a taurine deficiency should occur. Normally bile acids are deconjugated and reconjugated during enterohepatic cycling (Hofmann 1977b). In health, the amount of bile acids which are conjugated with glycine or taurine is probably 5–10 mmol/day, the majority of this being used for reconjugation of unconjugated bile acids returning from the intestine, and the minority being used for conjugation of frequently synthesized bile acids. In healthy persons, the amount of glycine and taurine used for total conjugation is probably 5–10 mmol/day (Hoffman and Hofmann 1974). In the patient with a biliary fistula the requirement for conjugation of newly synthesized bile acids increases 5- to 10-fold, as already noted. However, the requirement for reconjugation is eliminated. Hence the total amino acid required for conjugation should be similar in a healthy subject and a patient with a biliary fistula.

### *Indirect Effects*

Fat malabsorption has two major consequences (see Hofmann 1977c). The first is caloric deficiency, and its importance depends on the caloric requirement of the patient. Thus, fat malabsorption can be extremely important in the growing child and is often of no significance in the adult. The other consequence of fat malabsorption is due to the pharmacological effects of fatty acids in the colon. Here, they induce water and electrolyte secretion, and probably increase the permeability of the colon to anions which are not normally absorbed, such as oxalate.

Bile acids in the small intestine probably solubilize calcium which is complexed to the micelle (Moore et al. 1982). In the absence of bile acids, calcium soaps form and dietary oxalate now passes into solution, rather than being precipitated as an insoluble calcium salt (Smith and Hofmann 1974; Earnest 1979). As a consequence, oxalate enters the colon in solution, where, in the presence of malabsorbed fatty acids, altered colonic permeability permits the oxalate to be absorbed (Chadwick et al. 1973). Thus, it is entirely possible that a patient with a biliary fistula should have hyperoxaluria. However, in the absence of malabsorption of other anions, such as phosphate and sulfate, calcium activity in urine should probably remain low, and precipitation of calcium oxalate is unlikely to occur (Smith et al. 1980).

If bile acids are the body's natural cathartics, then in principle, a bile acid deficiency in the large intestine might cause constipation. However, since fatty acids are also secretory, such a problem should not occur. Unabsorbed fatty acids are converted by bacteria to hydroxy fatty acids, which mole for mole, are more potent secretagogues than dietary fatty acids. It must be emphasized that all long-chain fatty acids are secretory (Ammon and Phillips 1973).

## Treatment

Treatment depends on the nature of the problem. The first problem is whether fluid and electrolyte losses are sufficient to cause dehydration or electrolyte imbalance. If so, oral replacement of fluids should be possible. There is no reason why fluids cannot be given orally, and parenteral fluids should not be required unless the patient cannot take fluids orally. If there is a massive choleresis, somatostatin can be explored, since animal studies suggest that it inhibits ductular reabsorption (Rene et al. 1983). Fat malabsorption in the adult can be managed by a low-fat diet, with polyglucose supplements. In the child, medium-chain triglyceride supplementation may be necessary. In principle, there is no reason why pancreatic enzyme supplementation should be required.

Water-soluble derivatives of vitamin K should be given, and in instances of prolonged biliary drainage, 1,25 di-hydroxy vitamin $D_3$ may be given parenterally or the 25 hydroxy vitamin $D_3$ may be given orally (Long and Sherlock 1979). As noted, red blood cell morphology should be checked, and in instances of prolonged biliary drainage it may be desirable to measure the serum vitamin $B_{12}$ level.

In principle, bile flow should be of low viscosity and free of sludge. The current view is that sludge is composed of mucus and fibrin, together with some crystals of calcium bilirubinate. The unconjugated bilirubin is presumably formed by deconjugation somewhere in the ductular system (Boonyapisit et al. 1978).

In principle, one would think that bile flow should be kept as rapid as possible. Experiments proving therapeutic efficacy of choleretics have not been published. An additional problem is that choleretics which lower the micellar fraction of bile, i.e., which dilute bile, increase the cholesterol saturation of bile (Carey and Small 1978). Further, since the micelle probably complexes calcium, lowering the micellar fraction should increase calcium activity in bile, increasing the risk for precipitation of calcium salts, such as calcium bilirubinate or calcium carbonate. At the moment, the only choleretic with documented efficacy is dehydrocholate (Decholin), which is metabolized to non-micelle-forming bile acids (Soloway et al. 1973) and which, by virtue of its osmotic effect, induces a prompt choleresis. Perhaps therapeutic trials should be carried out with Decholin to determine whether its choleretic effect is of clinical utility.

Ursodeoxycholic acid is mildly choleretic in animals (Gilmore et al. 1982), but it is not known if it is choleretic in man.

## Epilogue

If internal drainage of the biliary tract by duct entero-stenting becomes the rule, then external biliary diversion will become an increasing rarity, or if it is seen, it will be only on a temporary basis. Based on current information, the major consequence of a biliary fistula is a bile acid deficiency in the small intestine which will cause triglyceride and fat-soluble malabsorption. Fluid replacement by animal bile salts, e.g. ox bile salts, should be efficacious, and if necessary, a low-fat diet or medium chain triglyceride can be explored. Fluid and electrolyte loss could be a problem in the rare patient, and somatostatin may help. A folic acid or vitamin $B_{12}$ deficiency is a theoretical possibility. Choleretics, such as Decholin, increase bile flow, but their clinical utility is unestablished. Finally, it must be emphasized that relatively little is known about the chemistry of bile, so that the possibility of a true bile loss syndrome involving biliary constituents not recognized at present always remains a possibility.

**Acknowledgements**

This work was supported in part by Research Grant AM 21506 from the National Institutes of Health and by grants-in-aid from the Falk Foundation and Stokely Van Camp, Inc.

**References**

Adlercreutz H, Martin F, Jarvenpaa P, Fotsis T (1979) Steroid absorption and enterohepatic recycling. Contraception 20:201–203
Ammon HV, Phillips SF (1973) Inhibition of colonic water and electrolyte absorption by fatty acids in man. Gastroenterology 65:744–749
Binder HJ, Filburn B, Floch M (1975) Bile acid inhibition of intestinal anaerobic organisms. Am J Clin Nutr 28:119–125
Bode JC, Zelder O, Bode C (1979) Qualitative and quantitative alterations of hepatic bile flow during recovery from extrahepatic cholestasis. In: Gentilini P, Popper H, Sherlock S, Teodori U (eds) Problems in intrahepatic cholestasis. Karger, Basel, pp 83–87
Boonyapisit ST, Trotman BW, Ostrow JD (1978) Unconjugated bilirubin, and the hydrolysis of conjugated bilirubin, in gallbladder bile of patients with cholelithiasis. Gastroenterology 74:70–74
Borgstrom B (1969) Quantification of cholesterol absorption in man by fecal analysis after the feeding of a single isotope-labeled meal. J Lipid Res 10:331–337
Carey MC (1979) Physical chemistry of bile: lipid solubility. In: Fisher MM, Goresky CA, Shaffer EA, Strasberg SM (eds) Gallstones. Plenum, New York, pp 131–141
Carey MC, Small DM (1978) The physical chemistry of cholesterol solubility in bile. J Clin Invest 61:998–1026
Chadwick VS, Modha K, Dowling RH (1973) Mechanism of hyperoxaluria in patients with ileal dysfunction. N Engl J Med 289:172–176
Colburn WA (1979) A pharmacokinetic model for enterohepatic circulation in the rat: phenolphthalein, a model drug. Drug Metab Dispos 7:100–102
Dowling RH, Mack E, Small DM (1970) Effects of controlled interruption of the enterohepatic circulation of bile salts by biliary diversion and by ileal resection on bile salt secretion, synthesis, and pool size in the Rhesus monkey. J Clin Invest 49:232–242
Dumont AE (1982) Significance of excess drainage of bile in patients with chronic hepatic disease. Surg Gynecol Obstet 154:209–213
Earnest DL (1979) Enteric hyperoxaluria. Adv Intern Med 24:407–427
Gilmore IT, LaRusso NF, Hofmann AF, Turcotte J, Carlson GL, Ott BJ (1982) Effects of individual taurine-conjugated bile acids on biliary secretion and sucrose clearance in the unanesthetized dog. Am J Physiol 5:G40–G46
Green R, Jacobsen DW, van Tonder SV, Kew MC, Metz J (1981) Enterohepatic circulation of cobalamin in the non-human primate. Gastroenterology 81:773–776
Hoffman NE, Hofmann AF (1974) Metabolism of steroid and amino acid moieties of conjugated bile acids in man. IV. Description and validation of a multicompartment model. Gastroenterology 67:887–897
Hofmann AF (1965) Clinical implications of physicochemical studies on bile salts. Gastroenterology 48:484–494
Hofmann AF (1977 a) Bile acids, diarrhea, and antibiotics: data, speculation, and a unifying hypothesis. J Infect Dis 135:S126–S136

Hofmann AF (1977b) The enterohepatic circulation of bile acids in man. Clin Gastroenterol 6:3–24
Hofmann AF (1977c) Malabsorption due to bile acid deficiency. In: Louhija A, Valtonen V (eds) Internal medicine 1976 topics. Karger, Basel, pp 18–28
Knoebel LK (1972) Intestinal absorption in vivo of micellar and nonmicellar lipids. Am J Physiol 223:255–261
Kumar R, Nagubandi S, Mattox VR, Londowski JM (1980) Enterohepatic physiology of 1, 25-dihydroxy vitamin $D_3$. J Clin Invest 65:277–284
Long RG, Sherlock S (1979) Vitamin D in chronic liver disease. Prog Liver Dis 6:539–555
Moore EW, Celic L, Ostrow JD Jr (1982) Interactions between $Ca^{++}$ and sodium taurocholate: bile salts are important buffers for prevention of calcium-containing gallstones. Gastroenterology 83:1079–1089
Owen CA Jr (1964) Absorption and excretion of $Cu^{64}$ labelled copper by the rat. Am J Physiol 207:1203–1206
Pertsemlidis D, Kirchman EH, Ahrens EH Jr (1973) Regulation of cholesterol metabolism in the dog. I. Effects of complete bile diversion and of cholesterol feeding on absorption, synthesis, accumulation, and excretion rates measured during life. J Clin Invest 52:2353–2367
Rene E, Danzinger RG, Hofmann AF, Nakagaki M (1983) The pharmacological effect of somatostatin on bile formation in the dog: enhanced ductular reabsorption as the major mechanism of anticholeresis. Gastroenterology 84:120–129
Rosenblum JL, Keating JP, Prensky AL, Nelson JS (1981) A progressive neurologic syndrome in children with chronic liver disease. N Engl J Med 304:503–508
Smith LH, Hofmann AF (1974) Acquired hyperoxaluria, urolithiasis, and intestinal disease: A new digestive disorder. Gastroenterology 66:1257–1261 (editorial)
Smith LH, Werness PG, Wilson DM, Phillips SF (1980) Enteric hyperoxaluria: Role of malabsorption of fluid and electrolytes in the formation of renal calculi. Clin Res 28:486A (abstract)
Soloway RD, Hofmann AF, Thomas PJ, Schoenfield LJ, Klein PD (1973) Triketocholanoic acid: hepatic metabolism and effect on bile flow and biliary lipid secretion in man. J Clin Invest 52:715–724
Steinberg SE, Campbell CL, Hillman RS (1979) Kinetics of the normal folate enterohepatic cycle. J Clin Invest 64:83–88
Tangedahl TN, Thistle JL, Hofmann AF, Matseshe JW (1979) Effect of $\beta$-sitosterol alone or in combination with chenic acid on the cholesterol saturation of bile and cholesterol absorption in gallstone patients. Gastroenterology 76:1341–1346
Thompson ABR, Dietschy JM (1981) Intestinal lipid absorption. In: Physiology of the Gastrointestinal Tract. LR Johnson, editor. Raven Press, New York, pp 1147–1220
Whipple GH (1965) Hemoglobin regeneration as influenced by diet and other factors. Nobel Lecture, 1934. In: Nobel Lectures Physiology or Medicine. Elsevier, Amsterdam, pp 346–353
Whipple GH, Hawkins WB (1935) Bile fistulas and related abnormalities. Bleeding, osteoporosis, cholelithiasis, and duodenal ulcers. J Exp Med 62:599–620